Global Health and Human Rights

This textbook explores public health and individual health care through the prism of global human rights and ethical decision-making.

Written by leading experts in this field, the book is divided into three distinctive parts. Part I introduces the theoretical framework through which the core issues can be understood, contrasting a clinical approach to health care with a social determinant perspective and discussing the decolonialisation of global health. Part II discusses how a human rights rationale impacts different social groups, from children to the elderly to those with disabilities, highlighting issues such as abortion and euthanasia. Part III addresses contemporary topics such as infectious diseases, migration, mental health care, the impact of advanced medical technology and climate change. Each chapter features case studies which ask readers to assess complex ethical dilemmas, fostering decision-making based on clear moral reasoning, as well as discussion assignments and further reading.

Also featuring online video lectures, this is an important textbook that will be essential reading for students across the health sciences, including medicine and all related fields.

Cees J. Hamelink is Athena Professor of Globalisation, Public Health and Human Rights at the Vrije Universiteit (VU) in Amsterdam, the Netherlands. He is Emeritus Professor of Communication Science at the University of Amsterdam and Emeritus Professor of Theology and Communication at the VU Amsterdam. He has published 21 academic monographs, and his most recent book (2023) is on communication and human rights.

Dirk R. Essink is Assistant Professor of Global Health at the Athena Institute, Vrije Universiteit Amsterdam, focusing on health systems and transdisciplinarity. His research, concentrated in Vietnam, Lao PDR, Ethiopia and South Sudan, explores the integration of knowledge for public health policy and transformations. Dirk's work emphasises social justice, covering quality of care in humanitarian settings, infectious disease control and sexual and reproductive health, nutrition and research agenda setting. He is skilled in transdisciplinary, mixed methods research.

Marlies J. Visser is a researcher and lecturer at the Athena Institute, Vrije Universiteit Amsterdam. She is an experienced qualitative researcher and in that capacity has coordinated and contributed to various research projects addressing social determinants of health and access to health care, with a particular emphasis on stigma and discrimination in relation to both physical and mental health conditions and sexual and reproductive health.

Global Health and Human Rights

Principles and Practices

Edited by
Cees J. Hamelink, Dirk R. Essink and
Marlies J. Visser

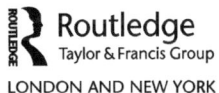

Routledge
Taylor & Francis Group

LONDON AND NEW YORK

Designed cover image: Getty images

First published 2025
by Routledge
4 Park Square, Milton Park, Abingdon, Oxon OX14 4RN

and by Routledge
605 Third Avenue, New York, NY 10158

Routledge is an imprint of the Taylor & Francis Group, an informa business

British Library Cataloguing-in-Publication Data
A catalogue record for this book is available from the British Library

ISBN: 978-1-032-52857-1 (hbk)
ISBN: 978-1-032-50374-5 (pbk)
ISBN: 978-1-003-40876-5 (ebk)

DOI: 10.4324/9781003408765

Typeset in Sabon
by Apex CoVantage, LLC

Access the Support Material: www.routledge.com/9781032503745

In 2008 the president of the Board of the Vrije Universiteit (VU), Prof. Dr Wim Noomen asked me whether I would be interested to teach human rights and health at the VU. Upon my positive answer I was contacted by Dr Joske Bunders, Professor of Biology and Society and Director of the Athena Institute at the VU. This encounter resulted in the plan for a course on globalisation, health and human rights and an Athena professorship.

When the course started around 2010 the angel that guarded the programme was Ms Anna van Luijn, who died much too early and to whom we want to dedicate this textbook. After each course iteration, Anna would say, "but we do not have a real textbook for the students".

Dear Anna, herewith we try to fulfil your wish!

Cees J. Hamelink

Contents

List of Figures and Tables	ix
List of Contributors	xi
List of Abbreviations	xv
Links to Online Video Resources	xvii

Introduction   1
Cees J. Hamelink, Dirk R. Essink and Marlies J. Visser

Part I   Introduction to Global Health and Human Rights   5

1   International Human Rights   7
Cees J. Hamelink

2   An Introduction to Global Health   27
Abdul K. Azad and Dirk R. Essink

3   The Right to Health   45
Cees J. Hamelink

4   Towards Human Rights Ethics: Marrying Intuitionism, Reasoning and Communication   65
Cees J. Hamelink

Part II   Health and Human Rights of Othered and Marginalised Groups   81

5   Sexual and Reproductive Health and Rights: A Perspective on Gender Bias and Stereotyping in Health   83
Marlies J. Visser

CONTENTS

6　Disability and Human Rights　　109
Mitzi M. Waltz

7　Mental Health and Psychiatric Care　　123
Miryam R. R. Holguín, Cees J. Hamelink and Tesania Velázquez

8　Children and the Right to Health　　135
Cees J. Hamelink and Victòria Fumadó

9　Elderly People and the Right to Health　　149
Cees J. Hamelink and Bert Keizer

10　Indigenous Peoples' Human Rights and Health　　161
Monserrat Vásquez Ladron de Guevara and Pilar M. d'Alò

Part III　Future Challenges in Global Health and Human Rights　　177

11　Public Health Emergencies, Pandemics and Human Rights　　179
Dirk R. Essink

12　Technology and the Right to Health　　201
Cees J. Hamelink and Dirk R. Essink

13　Planning for the Future　　209
Cees J. Hamelink, Dirk R. Essink and Marlies J. Visser

Epilogue　　217
Index　　219

Figures and Tables

Figures

2.1	Equality and Equity	33
2.2	Equality, Equity and Liberation Equality and Equity	34
2.3	Life Expectancy, 2021	37
2.4	Healthy Life Expectancy, 2019	37
2.5	Total Health Expenditure per Person, 2021	38
2.6	Share of Out-of-pocket Expenditure on Health Care, 2021	38
6.1a	The Medical Model of Disability	112
6.1b	The Social Model of Disability	113
6.2	Disability–poverty Vulnerability Cycle	116
13.1	Societal Determinants of Health in Policy vs Advancement of Medical Technology	213

Tables

6.1	Medical Model and Social Model	113

Contributors

Abdul K. Azad is Assistant Professor of Public Health and Human Development at O.P. Jindal Global University, India. He identifies as an activist scholar dedicated to transdisciplinary research and transformative practices through knowledge co-creation. His work centres around issues of epistemic justice, resilience and well-being. Currently, his work explores rights issues of statelessness among communities in Assam, India.

Pilar M. d'Alò is a doctoral researcher in political sociology at Newcastle University. Pilar's project interrogates the role of enduring colonial legacies of knowledge/power in Argentina by tracing the conditions of possibility for the making of "spiritual" as political in the Green Tide feminist movement. The project addresses contemporary issues over social movements, decolonisation and representation.

Dirk R. Essink is Assistant Professor of Global Health at the Athena Institute, Vrije Universiteit Amsterdam, focusing on health systems and transdisciplinarity. His research, concentrated in Vietnam, Lao PDR, Ethiopia and South Sudan, explores the integration of knowledge for public health policy and transformations. Dirk's work emphasises social justice, covering quality of care in humanitarian settings, infectious disease control and sexual and reproductive health, nutrition and research agenda setting. He is skilled in transdisciplinary, mixed methods research.

Victòria Fumadó is a paediatrician at the Hospital Sant Joan de Déu, Barcelona and Professor of Paediatrics at the University of Barcelona. She has dedicated her career to improving health care for children in humanitarian settings. She has been Founder and Director of Africa Viva Foundation since 1995. In that capacity she coordinates health training programs across Africa, specifically on nutrition and maternal health in fragile settings. More recently she has focussed on care for refugee children.

Cees J. Hamelink is Athena Professor of Globalisation, Health and Human Rights at the Athena Institute at the Vrije Universiteit (VU) Amsterdam. He is Emeritus Professor of Communication Science of the University of Amsterdam and Emeritus Professor of Theology and Communication of the VU Amsterdam. He has published 21 academic monographs. His most recent book (2023) is on communication and human rights with Polity Press.

Miryam R. R. Holguín is a professor at Pontifical Catholic University of Perú. Her research and practice focus on community psychology, emphasising human rights and mental health, public policies, emergencies and vulnerable contexts. She is an editorial board member of *INTERVENTION, the Journal of Mental Health and Psychosocial Support in Conflict Affected Areas*. She holds a PhD in psychology from the University of Leuven, Belgium.

Bert Keizer studied philosophy in England and medicine in Amsterdam, where he worked as a resident physician in nursing homes until 2015. Since then he has been active at the "Expertisecentrum Euthanasie" – a national organisation specialising in complex cases of euthanasia. He wrote books about his work in care for the elderly, about Wittgenstein, about the philosophical aspects of neurosurgery and about philosophy of mind, and he wrote the libretto for *The Alzheimer Opera*.

Monserrat Vásquez Ladron de Guevara (they/them) is a mestizo transdisciplinary artist, lecturer and researcher from Valparaíso, Chile. At the Vrije Universiteit Amsterdam, they focus on global health and environmental sciences, exploring the impact of Western colonial mechanisms on Indigenous livelihoods. Their doctoral research examines how colonial legacies, including forced resettlements and land grabbing, have affected Mapuche health, knowledge, identity and biodiversity. Using participatory and decolonial methods, Monserrat works with Indigenous communities to advocate for their rights and challenge dominant narratives, aiming to enhance understanding of Indigenous experiences and justice.

Tesania Velázquez earned her doctorate in psychology from the Pontificia Universidad Católica del Perú (PUCP) and her master's in clinical and forensic evaluation from the University of Salamanca, Spain. She is a professor at the department of psychology and at the master's degree program in community psychology at PUCP. She works in the research lines of forensic psychology, penitentiary psychology, intervention in post-disaster contexts, gender violence and community psychology.

Marlies J. Visser is a researcher and lecturer at the Athena Institute, Vrije Universiteit Amsterdam. She is an experienced qualitative researcher and in that capacity has coordinated and contributed to various research projects addressing social determinants of health and access to health care, with a particular emphasis on stigma and discrimination in relation to both physical and mental health conditions and sexual and reproductive health.

Mitzi M. Waltz is Program Coordinator of the Research Master Global Health and has dedicated her career to fostering inclusion for people with disabilities globally. Her work includes collaborating on research with disabled individuals, developing an inclusion-focused workforce, addressing health care disparities and shaping policy. With over 30 years of experience as a researcher, journalist and media educator, she is committed to furthering the rights of people living with disabilities.

Abbreviations

AAAQ	Available, accessible, acceptable and of good quality
ABR	Adolescent birth rate
AI	Artificial intelligence
AIIHPH	All India Institute of Hygiene and Public Health
AU	African Union
CDC	Centre of Disease Control
CEDAW	Convention on the Elimination of Discrimination Against Women
CRPD	Convention on the Rights of Persons with Disabilities
CSW	Commission on the Status of Women
DPO	Disabled People's Organisation
ECOSOC	Economic and Social Council of the UN
EMRIP	Expert mechanisms on the rights of Indigenous peoples
EU	European Union
FAO	Food and Agriculture Organization of the United Nations
GBV	Gender-based violence
GDP	Gross domestic product
HIC	High-income countries
HRE	Human rights education
IACHR	Inter-American Commission on Human Rights
ICCPR	International Covenant on Civil and Political Rights
ICESCR	International Covenant on Economic, Social and Cultural Rights
ICF	International classification of functioning, disability and health
ICPD	International Conference on Population and Development
ICT	Information communication technology
IHR	International health regulations
ILO	International Labour Organisation

IMF	International Monetary Fund
IWGIA	International Work Group for Indigenous Affairs
LGBTQI	Lesbian gay bisexual transgender queer and intersex
LMIC	Low- and middle-income countries
MMR	Maternal mortality ratio
NCDs	Non-communicable diseases
OHCHR	Office of the High Commissioner for Human Rights
OP	Optional protocol
PHEIC	Public health emergency of international concern
PoA	Programme of action
RCT	Randomised controlled trial
SARS	Severe acute respiratory syndrome
SDGs	Sustainable Development Goals
SDH	Social determinants of health
SIM	Social intuitionist model
SRH	Sexual and reproductive health
SRHR	Sexual and reproductive health and rights
TB	Tuberculosis
UDHR	Universal Declaration of Human Rights
UHC	Universal health coverage
UK	United Kingdom
UN	United Nations
UN DESA	UN Department of Economic and Social Affairs
UNDRIP	UN Declaration on the Rights of Indigenous Peoples
UNICEF	United Nations Children's Fund
UNFPA	United Nations Population Fund
US	United States of America
VU	Vrije Universiteit Amsterdam
WHO	World Health Organisation

Links to Online Video Resources

Chapter 1: On Human Rights
https://www.kaltura.com/index.php/extwidget/preview/partner_id/1197662/uiconf_
    id/46402141/entry_id/1_r9cdirzu/embed/iframe?
Chapter 3: On Human Rights and Health
https://www.kaltura.com/index.php/extwidget/preview/partner_id/1197662/uiconf_
    id/46402141/entry_id/1_bsxsnlei/embed/iframe?
Chapter 7: On Human Rights and Mental Health
https://www.kaltura.com/index.php/extwidget/preview/partner_id/1197662/uiconf_
    id/46402141/entry_id/1_hzm7wuh9/embed/iframe?
Chapter 9: On Human Rights and Elderly Care
https://www.kaltura.com/index.php/extwidget/preview/partner_id/1197662/uiconf_
    id/46402141/entry_id/1_fgsuo50w/embed/iframe?
Chapter 10: On Human Rights and Indigenous People
https://www.kaltura.com/index.php/extwidget/preview/partner_id/1197662/uiconf_
    id/46402141/entry_id/1_3b2cygrk/embed/iframe?
Chapter 11: On Human Rights and Pandemics
https://www.kaltura.com/index.php/extwidget/preview/partner_id/1197662/uiconf_
    id/46402141/entry_id/1_q04yf51w/embed/iframe?

Introduction

Cees J. Hamelink, Dirk R. Essink and Marlies J. Visser

This textbook is based upon the MSc-level course Global Health and Human Rights that we teach at the Athena Institute of the Vrije Universiteit in Amsterdam. The course has a strong emphasis on the ambition to achieve the "highest attainable standard of health" (expressed in several United Nations human rights instruments). According to a General Comment (no. 14) of the Office of the UN High Commissioner for Human Rights (OHCHR), this standard implies that health care is available, accessible, acceptable and of good quality (AAAQ) to ensure the enjoyment of health for all people, without any form of discrimination. Health care must include children as well as older people, people with disabilities, women and girls seeking sexual and reproductive health care, Indigenous peoples and those requiring psychiatric care, for example. In the daily praxis of health care, challenges may arise, such as denial of access to certain health services or the imposition of coercive procedures or treatments against the will of individuals treating them as passive objects rather than autonomous beings. In addition, instances occur where human rights are in conflict with other pressing issues such as the protection of people's health during pandemics or situations in which using advanced medical technology to improve effectivity and efficiency of health care services collides with individual rights to the protection of privacy. As in reality, violations of basic principles of human rights such as autonomy, dignity, equality and security persist across all levels of society; the course examines infringements of human rights that occur in relation to the provision of adequate health care, the decision-making procedures in health care and the institutional infrastructures involved.

Following our course outline, the textbook thematically explores and discusses important dimensions of global health and health care in the light of human rights. During the course we address the various challenges marginalised and "othered" individuals, groups and communities can experience to achieve the "highest attainable standard of health" and the complex dilemmas that may arise in safeguarding the right to health. In the book we also draw attention to the complementarity of human rights and human responsibilities.

DOI: 10.4324/9781003408765-1

The textbook puts health issues in a contemporary historical context and invites discussions on how the prevailing international order can accommodate the requirements of the human right to health. The book covers various topics in global health and human rights and is divided over three distinctive parts:

- Part I of the book connects health to human rights in a global context. This part introduces and connects international human rights, global health and the human right to health. Further, it introduces a human rights method of ethics.
- Part II of the book discusses various key themes within global health and human rights and the in- and exclusion of "othered" groups following the human rights framework. This part engages with the realities in health and health care of various marginalised groups and communities and discusses some of the complex dilemmas that may arise in ensuring the human rights principles of autonomy, dignity, equality and security.
- Part III of the book addresses contemporary issues in health and human rights which pose significant challenges to the future of health and human rights. We selected two key future challenges to discuss in the book: future infectious diseases and global pandemics and the development of medical technology. The book concludes with a chapter on planning for the future and introduces a practical instrument following scenario development that readers may use when thinking about the future of global health and human rights.

Throughout the book, we explore and connect macro frameworks, meso-level contexts and micro-level experiences to provide a comprehensive analysis of human rights violations in global health. We aim to offer a broad understanding of the complexities and challenges in promoting human rights in health. We acknowledge that this book provides a non-exhaustive introduction to key challenges in global health and human rights. Our focus is on topics that we believe have a significant impact on daily health care practices. Chapters are written by teachers in the course and invited specialists in the different fields. Some chapters include additional mini-lectures provided through short video clips. Each chapter includes a set of discussion questions, encouraging readers to reflect on the principles and practices covered in the chapter.

For Whom Did We Write This Textbook?

This textbook is primarily intended as a guide for students and practitioners in health sciences, medicine and related fields, providing essential knowledge and insights into the significance of and challenges to human rights-based health care. Its primary aim is to introduce human rights in health, encouraging critical thinking on key issues in global health and human rights. By exploring health and health care practices grounded in the human right to health, readers will engage with complex dilemmas. To support students' critical thinking and analysis, the book offers practical tools making it an invaluable resource for those committed to advancing equitable health care.

How to Read This Textbook

In the course of the textbook, students will be invited to critically reflect on and exercise cases of contextual ethics in health and health care. The book aspires to provide students with some key topical background knowledge as well as guidance for ways and methods of dealing with complex dilemmas. In the daily practice of health care, numerous decisions have to be made in real time. From professionals it may be expected that they are capable of accounting for the choices they make. Essential choices in health care require the development of professional moral reasoning. We have added a novel approach to moral choice in health care: a human rights method of ethics.

In this book the focus is on the permanent interaction between principles and choice situations. From this it can be learned how different contexts create new perspectives on basic principles as social instruments that evolve in interaction with different concrete situations. The international human rights framework is constituted by the norms embedded in the instruments that the international community has formally accepted. The question is how this framework can be applied to concrete daily practice in global health and health care.

Throughout the textbook, we use the notion of human rights and deliberately do not use concepts like basic rights, civic rights or constitutional rights. The working of these rights is often restricted to citizens of national states, and human rights is the broader, all-inclusive normative standard. We were guided by the essential declaration that "all people matter".

The textbook proposes that moral issues should be resolved within the complexity of concrete historical, cultural, professional and institutional circumstances. This requires a process of dialogical moral reasoning that begins casuistically with an understanding of what moral issue is at stake and with questioning the institutional settings and professional network-relations in which the issue is located. Questions are asked about the consequences of different choices and the dialogue moves back and forth between general (human rights) principles and the details of the issue at stake. The authors have chosen a case-driven approach to the challenging encounter of health practices with human rights standards. Dialogical moral reasoning assists the fine-tuning of the capacity and the sensitivity for moral arguments. It is a mutual learning exercise. In the process stakeholders learn from the other, listen to the other and try to understand the perspective of the other. The attempt to understand different moral premises and conclusions may inspire mutual respect rather than unproductive disagreement. Dialogical reasoning needs to be learned! This textbook aspires to make a contribution to this learning process.

Introduction to Global Health and Human Rights

Part I introduces the main concepts that underpin this book: global health, the human rights framework, the right to health and contextual ethics. In the first chapter, we define global health and explain how it is related to human rights and how our health systems aim to contribute to a state of "complete physical, social and mental well-being". However, not all benefit equally from health care, and inequities persist. Moreover, the way we practice global health may actually reproduce these inequities.

In the second chapter, the origins and philosophical underpinnings of the human rights framework are presented along with how these contributed to the drafting of the Universal Declaration of Human Rights (1948). We discuss the significance and universality of this human rights declaration and go into the some of the complexities that may arise in enforcing human rights.

In the third chapter, we bring together the concepts of global health and human rights. We unpack the right to health and social conditionalities of health, address the institutionalisation of health care, the role of the UN Special Rapporteurs on the Right to Health and the need for human rights education. In this chapter, we emphasise how contextual ethics, guided by human rights principles of dignity, autonomy, equality and security, contribute to a human rights-based approach to health care.

In the fourth chapter, we explore a human rights-based approach to the moral choices that have to be made in health care and in the management of health care institutions.

DOI: 10.4324/9781003408765-2

International Human Rights

Cees J. Hamelink

Introduction

International human rights form a regulatory framework with legal and moral rules for human behaviour and institutions for their implementation. The framework sets international standards and has the function to promote, implement and enforce these standards. Today its key institutional basis are the United Nations (UN), both the author of essential human rights instruments (declarations, resolutions, treaties) and an association of some of the worst human rights violators. The promotion of human rights is most forcefully exercised by non-governmental organisations such as the International Federation of Human Rights (established in 1922), Amnesty International, Human Rights Watch and numerous smaller organisations that defend the interests of children, women, Indigenous peoples, sexual minorities, refugees and people with disabilities. Implementation is largely left to institutions on the regional and national level, such as the European Court of Human Rights or the Inter-American Court of Human Rights. By and large the global implementation and enforcement of human rights standards is very weak. A key obstacle to the implementation and enforcement is the inherent tension among the key concepts of international law, "state sovereignty", and universal human rights. The implementation of human rights by the UN and national governments is highly politicised. The drafting of the Universal Declaration of Human Rights was a process of political agreements and disagreements.

At its core, the human rights framework addresses an issue that can be found in many cultures throughout the ages: the abuse of power. The human rights framework is intended primarily to protect individuals from the abuse of power by governments, governmental agencies, judiciary institutions, corporate entities and powerful individuals. The notions of power and abuse of power date way back in human history and are universal.

The key philosophical problem of human rights is their justification. Why should we have human rights? The justification question is in fact the old theme of moral philosophy: why should I be moral?

DOI: 10.4324/9781003408765-3

In this chapter we explore how far human rights make sense in relation to issues of global health. In exploring an answer, we shall see that understanding human rights is a matter of transdisciplinary studies. It involves ethics, philosophy, law, history, politics, political economy, development economics, conflict studies, sociology, anthropology and social psychology.

Learning Objectives
After studying this chapter unit you will be able to:

■ Explain the development of the international human rights framework
■ Challenge and defend the significance of the international human rights framework
■ Understand the obligations of states under international human rights law
■ Identify the major obstacles to the realisation of human rights
■ Discuss the conflicts between human rights and other pressing interests

The Development of the Human Rights Framework
The human species does not distinguish itself by a historical record that radiates benignity. Throughout most of its history, human beings occupied themselves with an impressive variety of humiliating acts against fellow human beings. Against this gross indecency of human history, the more enlightened individuals have throughout the ages committed themselves to the articulation and codification of basic moral standards that were intended to restrain human aggression, arbitrariness and negligence. Basic to the concept of human rights is the notion that the human being is entitled to respect for his or her inalienable dignity. This means that the human being is worthy of treatment in accordance with certain basic standards. The recognition of the dignity of the human person implies that human beings cannot treat each other arbitrarily in ways they see fit.

The standards of human conduct have evolved in a long history of different schools of religious and philosophical thought. The modern notion of human rights has many parents. Among them are those European thinkers who developed the idea of natural rights that became so central to political thinking from the 18th-century Enlightenment period onward. Liberal theories on natural rights articulated such rights in universal terms as rights by birth belonging to all people because they are human beings. For example, one finds this in the thinking of John Locke (1632–1704), who proposed that individuals are born free and equal and are endowed with natural rights in virtue of their common humanity. Yet, Locke excluded from these natural rights women and slaves, and from his right to religious tolerance he excluded Catholics and atheists. The modern idea that human rights are a reflection of universal moral principles was strongly influenced by the thinking of Immanuel Kant (1724–1804). Kant proposed that individuals can act autonomously and in accordance with reason. They can choose to act in accordance with universal moral principles. Such principles can be derived from reason. People can develop – when they distance themselves from their individual desires and interests – moral rules that would be freely adopted by all people under the same conditions. Universal moral rules imply moral obligations that are unconditional to all.

The primary moral obligation is that I should act in such a way that I can want my normative standard to become a universal law.

The secondary moral obligation is to always act in such a way that no individual is treated as a means to an end. The underlying notion is that the dignity of all individuals should be respected.

Such humanist conceptions also have many non-Western antecedents. The notion of human beings as rights bearers – which reflects a basic respect for human dignity and a tradition of tolerance, freedom and compassion – did not emerge from one single cultural source. It is a strange and unwarranted underestimation of non-Western cultural traditions to assume that only the West could have come up with a defence of the inherent dignity of all human beings. Actually, the West has been as much a place where ideas about rights to freedom, equality and democracy developed as it was the arena of slavery, racism, sexism and fascism.

As UN Secretary General Kofi Annan stated in a speech in 1997, "The principles enshrined in the Universal Declaration of Human Rights are deeply rooted in the history of humankind. They can be found in the teachings of all the world's cultural and religious traditions". The novelty of the international human rights framework – as it was established after 1945 – is the formulation of these principles as universal moral standards that were new for all parties in the international community. Human rights confront not only non-Western cultures with a historically new situation: they are a new and difficult challenge for all cultures. No culture, religion or moral system knows a set of rights and duties such as developed in the Universal Declaration of Human Rights (UDHR). In the declaration, in contrast to most cultural and religious traditions, the recognition of human dignity is formulated as a claim to be enforced by law. Moreover, this claim recognises that the individual is entitled to rights not only through membership of a community but in his or her own individual capacity.

Before 1945, there were human rights declarations such as the Magna Carta of 1215, the British Bill of Rights (1689), the American Declaration of Independence (1776) and the French Déclaration des droits de l'homme et du citoyen (1789). In 1945, this long history of the protection of human dignity acquired a fundamentally new significance. In the first place, the protection of human dignity (earlier mainly a national affair) was put on the agenda of the world community. Thus, the defence of fundamental rights was no longer the exclusive preoccupation of national politics and became an essential part of world politics. The judgement of whether human rights had been violated was no longer the exclusive monopoly of national governments. Earlier concerns about what happened in foreign countries were largely dependent on whether this affected one's politico-economic interests. Such concerns may have been whether one's diplomats would be treated correctly by other countries. There were no standards to treat all human beings decently. There was little or no altruism involved. International concerns were selective and did not imply compassion with humanity as such. Minority treaties under the League of Nations had little to do with respect for rights of minorities but were inspired by concerns about peace among nations. The unfair treatment of minorities could lead to disturbance of the peace. Concern for citizens of other states was hindered by strict conceptions of state sovereignty – but also by inadequate information. Moreover, how could states have intervened in other countries, whereas in most countries governments routinely violated those rights that later came to be called human rights? In the second place, the enjoyment of human rights was no longer restricted to privileged individuals and social elites. The revolutionary core of the process that began at San Francisco – with the adoption of the UN Charter in 1945 – is that "all people matter". There are no longer nonpersons. Basic rights hold for everyone and exclude no one. The American Declaration of Independence (1776) stated that individuals have inalienable rights that were subsequently recognised in the US Constitution and the Bill of Rights (1789). Slaves were excluded from these rights. Although there were many demands for its abolition (e.g., by Thomas Paine), slavery was only abolished in 1865. Also, women were excluded. The right to vote was only extended to women in 1920.

The French Déclaration excluded women, although there were strong demands for equal rights of women at the time. Among the protesting voices was Olympe de Gouge, who issued in 1790 The Declaration of the Rights of Women. The French National Assembly of 1792 refused this declaration. Olympe de Gouge was executed. Vincent Ogé pleaded for rights for mulattos – a now outdated and contested term that refers to people of mixed African and European ancestry – and their inclusion in the National Assembly at Paris. He was executed. It should also be remembered that the American and French declarations of human rights were written at the time of Western colonialism, and they had no provisions for people under colonial rule. In the third place, the conventional view that individuals can only be objects of international law changed to the conception that the individual is a holder of rights and bearer of duties under international law. The individual can appeal to international law for the protection of his or her rights but can also be held responsible for violations of human rights standards. The recognition of individual rights under international law was thus linked with the notion that individuals also have duties under international law. This was eloquently expressed in 1947 by Mahatma Gandhi in a letter to the director of UNESCO about the issue of human rights. Gandhi wrote, "I learnt from my illiterate but wise mother that rights to be deserved and preserved came from duty well done".

Most important, human rights standards propose that the moral claims that people make vis-à-vis each other are solely based on their humanity. If rights are related to the human being as such and not given by an authority, they cannot be taken away by whatever authority. They do not have to be deserved. They are not dependent on good conduct or divine grace. They are inherent to the human being because he or she is human. International human rights standards are grounded in the conviction that all human beings have inalienable entitlements to the protection of their life and liberty because of their humanity and not as derivatives of a higher order. This notion of human autonomy is certainly not universally shared. If progress is to be made in the implementation of human rights standards, we should get away from the common and convenient approach in which human rights are seen as mainly a problem for non-Western civilisations. It needs to be recognised that this denies that the West has great difficulties with the theory and practice of human rights. The human rights regime challenges fundamental ways of thinking in all cultural traditions. It reflects a mode of thought that is new to all societies, not just non-Western societies. There is widespread unwillingness to take human rights seriously in the East, West, North and South. For most communities around the world (whatever their cultural backgrounds), there are serious difficulties in grounding human rights. Human rights pose essential challenges to a Chinese Confucian culture but equally to a Western consumer culture, to Islamic as well as to Christian theology. The need for an internal critical discourse on human rights standards is equally strong everywhere.

Immediately after World War II, the international community, as it established the United Nations (UN) (in 1945), pointed at human rights as essential building blocks for the effort to realise a peaceful world. When in 1945 the Charter of the UN was adopted in San Francisco (UN, 1945), several member states urged that a Bill of Rights should be included in the document. This did not happen, but it was agreed to establish a Commission on Human Rights, which was to prepare an International Bill of Human Rights for the General Assembly.

The UN Charter made explicit reference to human rights in its Preamble and Articles 1, 13, 55, 56, 62 and 68. It stated herewith that human rights are seen as integral to the mandate and mission of the UN. Its visionary drafters expressed their fundamental conviction that the respect for human rights would be basic to international peace and development.

Following the UN Charter, human rights standards have been formulated in the so-called International Bill of Rights, which consists of the Universal Declaration of Human Rights (UDHR) (adopted on December 10, 1948, by the UN General Assembly) and the two key human rights treaties, the International Covenant on Economic, Social and Cultural Rights (ICSECR) (adopted in 1966 and in force since January 3, 1976) and the International Covenant on Civil and Political Rights (ICCPR) (adopted in 1966 and in force since March 23, 1976). Different dimensions of human rights have also been codified in a series of international treaties, in regional instruments (such as the European Convention for the Protection of Human Rights and Fundamental Freedoms (1950), the American Convention of Human Rights (1969), the African Charter on Human and Peoples' Rights (1981) and the Islamic Declaration of Human Rights, which was prepared by the Islamic Council 1980 and presented to UNESCO in 1981).

The documents (often called instruments) in which human rights are formulated have different legal meanings. In international relations, rules and practices among states can over time be accepted as international custom and, as such, become a source of international law. Increasingly, however, such customary law is replaced by conventions or treaties that have become the essential instruments of international cooperation. Treaties impose binding obligations on the parties who ratify them, which means making them officially valid. Often treaties are preceded by international declarations, which may have a strong moral impact (such as is the case with the Universal Declaration of Human Rights) but do not have a legally binding character. In addition to treaties and declarations, the international community can also recommend certain types of action through resolutions of its decision-making bodies such as the General Assembly of the UN. The essential instrument in the field of human rights remains the 1948 UDHR. The declaration continues to be a source of inspiration for thought and action in the field of human rights. The UDHR, although not a binding treaty, carries important legal weight. Among legal scholars there is a considerable consensus that the UDHR constitutes binding law as international custom. The Declaration is certainly recognised by civilised nations as a common and binding standard of achievement. The text proclaims a fairly comprehensive set of rights (and puts civil and political rights on the same level as social, economic and cultural rights) and also proposes the implementation of these claims in a social and international order.

The Universal Declaration of Human Rights

This first part of the declaration begins with reference to the recognition of human dignity: "whereas recognition of the inherent dignity and of the equal and inalienable rights of all members of the human family is the foundation of freedom, justice and peace in the world". The notion human dignity is not without difficulties, and its grounding is seriously contested in religion and philosophy.

A special problem is that human dignity tends to be defined in terms of the substantially superior nature of the human being in comparison with all other beings in the universe. To a large extent this justifies questionable human conduct regarding nonhuman forms of life such as animals. Human dignity remains a vague notion and yet it provides the grounds for freedom, justice and peace.

The barbarous acts of World War II are seen as resulting from a disregard for human rights. In the second paragraph of the Preamble, we find the four freedoms that President Franklin D. Roosevelt spoke about in his 1941 Message to the US Congress.

> Whereas disregard and contempt for human rights have resulted in barbarous acts which have outraged the conscience of mankind, and the advent of a world in which human beings shall enjoy freedom of speech and belief and freedom from fear and want has been pro-claimed as the highest aspiration of the common people.

The Preamble points to the international dimension of human rights and the key mission of the UN with this phrase: "whereas it is essential to promote the development of friendly relations between nations".

The Preamble confirms the commitment of the peoples of the UN to the defence of human rights and uses the following phrasing:

> whereas the peoples of the United Nations have in the Charter reaffirmed their faith in fundamental human rights, in the dignity and worth of the human person and in the equal rights of men and women and have determined to promote social progress and better standards of life in larger freedom, Whereas Member States have pledged themselves to achieve, in co-operation with the United Nations, the promotion of universal respect for and observance of human rights and fundamental freedoms.

It is important to note that the text states that protection by law is essential for human rights: "whereas it is essential, if man is not to be compelled to have recourse, as a last resort, to rebellion against tyranny and oppression, that human rights should be protected by the rule of law".

The Preamble continues with the observation that the implementation of human rights will, to a large extent, depend on the creation of a common worldwide understanding of what human rights are: "whereas a common understanding of these rights and freedoms is of the greatest importance for the full realisation of this pledge".

The Human Rights Standards

A common distinction among the rights and freedoms that form the core of international human rights standards refers to three generations of human rights. According to this division, civil and political rights (sometimes referred to as the classic human rights) are seen as the first generation. Economic, social and cultural rights make up the second generation and a series of collective rights form the third generation. The latter include the right to development, the right to peace and the right to a clean, natural environment. As Baehr (1999) rightly remarked

> The term "generations" is somewhat unfortunate. It suggests a succession of phenomena, whereby a new generation takes the place of the previous one. That is, however, not the case with the three "generations" of human rights. On the contrary. The idea is rather that the three "generations" exist and be respected simultaneously.
>
> *(p. 7)*

In the International Bill of Rights alone we find 76 different human rights. In the totality of major international and regional human rights instruments, this number is even greater. With the tendency among human rights lobbies to put more and more social problems in a human rights framework, the number of human rights is likely to further increase. Because this proliferation of rights does not necessarily strengthen the cause of the actual implementation of human rights, various attempts have been made to establish a set of core human rights that are representative for the totality. One effort concluded in the existence of 12 core rights (Jongman & Schmidt, 1994):

1. The right not to be discriminated against
2. The right to education
3. The right to political participation
4. The right to fair working conditions
5. The right to life
6. The right not to be tortured
7. The right not to be arbitrarily arrested
8. The right to food
9. The right to health care
10. The right to freedom of association
11. The right to political participation
12. The right to freedom of expression

These rights are the legal articulation of some underlying moral principles and their implied standards of human conduct. These basic principles and their related norms are:

- **Dignity** and the implied norm that acts of humiliation are not allowed.
- **Equality** and the implied norm that discrimination – on any grounds – is inadmissible. This principle entitles human beings to equal entitlement of fundamental resources, such as clean water, to equal participation in political decision-making and to equal treatment in terms of personal dignity.
- **Liberty** and the implied norm that obstruction of human self-determination inadmissible. This principle protects the autonomy of the human being.
- **Security** and the implied norm that intentional harm against human integrity is inadmissible. This principle proposes a standard of conduct against attacks upon people's physical, mental and moral integrity. It protects people against arbitrary

interference with their private sphere and against unlawful attacks on their honour and reputation. Example: some medical interventions may cause considerable harm to patients (like when limbs have to be amputated), and therefore these interventions may only take place with the informed consent of the patient.

The Mechanisms of Enforcement

No effective mechanism for the enforcement of human rights has been realised. This is unfortunate because for the protection of human rights the notion that there can be no rights without the option of redress in case of their violation is crucial. Rights and remedies are intrinsically related. Where human rights instruments do not provide accessible and affordable means of redress, they erode the effective protection of the rights they proclaim. The old adage of Roman law states, "ubi ius, ibi remedium" – where there is law, there is remedy. One can turn this around and propose that, when no remedy is available, there is no law. People should be able to seek effective remedy when state or private parties violate their human rights. Human rights not only require mechanisms of redress. They also imply that those who rule on behalf of others are accountable (i.e., they are obliged to justify their decisions on behalf of others). It is a basic requirement of human rights standards that provisions on public policy imply a mechanism for accountability. "The requirement that every citizen has a right to take part in the conduct of public affairs is satisfied if appointed officials are in some way responsible to elected representatives" (Partsch, 1981, p. 239). The realisation of human rights requires limitations on the power of the state as well as a defence against horizontal abuses of fundamental rights and freedoms. People should have access to effective redress when private actors interfere with their privacy, distribute misleading information or threaten their cultural autonomy.

On the basis of these principles (effective remedy, accountability and horizontal effect), the procedures for individuals and communities to seek redress have to contain at least the following three components.

First, the recognition of the formal right to file complaints in case public or private actors do not comply with the adopted standards.

Second, the recognition of the competence of an independent tribunal that receives complaints from both state and nonstate actors, individuals and communities.

Third, the recognition that the opinions of the tribunal are binding on those who accept its jurisdiction. Present remedial procedures are mainly based on the Optional Protocol (OP) to the International Covenant on Civil and Political Rights (1966) and Resolution 1503 adopted by the Economic and Social Council of the UN (ECOSOC) in 1970. The protocol authorises the UN Human Rights Committee to receive and consider communications from individuals subject to its jurisdiction who claim to be victims of a violation by that State Party of any of the rights set forth in the covenant. Individual complaints can only come from nationals of states that are party to the OP (presently 75 states). The OP provides for communications, analysis and reporting but not for sanctions. Resolution 1503 recognises the possibility of individual complaints about human rights violations. It authorises the UN Human Rights Commission to examine "communications, together with replies of governments, if any, which appear to reveal a consistent pattern of gross violations of human rights". The 1503 procedure is slow and confidential and provides individuals with no redress. Other institutional mechanisms for implementation in addition to the UN Commission on Human Rights are the

Human Rights Committee to Monitor the ICCPR; the Committee on the Elimination of Racial Discrimination; the Committee on Economic; Social and Cultural Rights; the Committee on the Elimination of Discrimination Against Women; the Committee Against Torture and the Committee on the Rights of the Child. However important these bodies' work is, their powers to enforce human rights standards are limited.

The UN Commission on Human Rights is a permanent body of the Economic and Social Council of the UN (ECOSOC). Its members are state representatives. Findings of the Commission have a certain significance but are not binding.

The Human Rights Committee consists of 18 experts supervising the implementation of the ICCPR. The work of the Committee covers only parties that ratified the covenant (presently 148 states) and provides international monitoring on the basis of reports provided by states. The Committee's monitoring does not imply any sanctions, but it can generate some negative publicity on a country's human rights performance.

For the implementation of the Race Convention, the Committee on the Elimination of Racial Discrimination has been established. The Committee can receive complaints from states, but only 14 states authorise the Committee to receive communications from individuals.

The implementation body for the 1979 Convention on the Elimination of Discrimination Against Women is the Committee on the Elimination of Discrimination Against Women. Since 1999, an Optional Protocol to the Convention makes it possible for the committee to process individual complaints.

The committee that examines the implementation of the Convention on the Rights of the Child does not have the authority to receive individual complaints.

The Committee on Economic, Social and Cultural Rights has no right to receive complaints from individuals or groups. In its submission to the 1993 UN World Conference on Human Rights, the committee argued for a formal complaints procedure in stating:

> as long as the majority of the provisions of the Covenant (and most notably those relating to education, health care, food and nutrition, and housing) are not subject of any detailed jurisprudential scrutiny at the international level, it is most unlikely that they will be subject to such examination at the national level either.
> *(UN Committee on Economic, Social and*
> *Cultural Rights, 1993, p. 92)*

In 1997, the 53rd session of the UN Commission on Human Rights discussed a draft protocol for a complaints procedure and affirmed in a resolution the interest of its members for the draft. This was the first step in the long process towards an optional protocol. International human rights law remains a weak and largely nonenforceable arrangement. It should not be ignored that this is a conscious political choice. Most nation-states have shown little interest in interference with their human rights record. The state-centric arrangement of world politics, in which states are unwilling to yield power over their citizens, is still dominant and stands squarely in the way of universal respect for human rights. In current world politics, states still maintain a considerable measure of sovereignty in the treatment of their citizens. Yet the UN World Conference on Human Rights of 1993 has reaffirmed that "the promotion and protection of all human rights is a legitimate concern of the international community". If indeed the most important issue for the significance and validity of the human rights framework is the implementation of the standards it proposes, the present worldwide lack of implementation of human rights standards poses the most serious challenge to the human rights regime. There is abundant evidence that human rights standards around the world are almost incessantly violated by actors with different political and ideological viewpoints. Usually in wars of liberation, for example, one finds gross violations by the hands of both the oppressors and the liberators. However, it is obvious that the world would be a different and far more humane place for many people if human rights standards were respected. If one studies the annual reports from such bodies as Amnesty International, there appear to be no countries where human rights are not violated. For moral philosophers, this is actually not a terribly surprising problem. It represents the classic gap between the moral knowledge human beings possess and their intention to act morally.

State Obligations

Under international human rights law, state-parties to human rights conventions have three types of obligation: the obligation to respect, to protect and to fulfil. Respect means that states should treat all persons in accordance with the fundamental rights to dignity, equality and freedom. It also means that states should not deprive persons of these rights. Protect means states should prevent the violation of these rights by non-state actors. Fulfil means states should adopt legislative, judiciary and budgetary measures towards the progressive realisation of these rights. The principle of "progressive realisation" is formulated in the International Covenant on Economic, Social and Cultural Rights (Article 2) as obligation for the state to take steps "to the maximum of its available resources". Crucially, because human rights are universal, states' obligations extend beyond their borders.

The Obstacles

There are several obstacles to the implementation of human rights.

Limited Visions on Human Rights

There are two prominent visions on human rights that hinder an effective implementation of human rights. The first vision perceives human rights almost exclusively as civil and political rights. The second vision focuses almost exclusively on relations between states and citizens.

The first vision. The almost exclusive perception of human rights as civil and political rights creates explosive contradictions between political conditionalities that press for good governance, democracy and respect for human rights and economic conditions that impose such austere measures that the resulting inequalities can only be controlled by highly undemocratic policies. The policies of the International Monetary Fund (IMF) have – across the Global South – undermined the economic conditions for democracy, such as education, social equality and reduction of poverty. The structural adjustment programs of the IMF in many countries weakened the capacity of governments to meet international human rights obligations. The neglect of basic social and economic rights undermines such civil and political rights as freedom of expression and freedom of association.

The second vision. This limited vision on human rights focuses on the vertical "state to citizen" relation and provides no legal force for human rights in horizontal relations such as between individuals (for example in the family: parent–child relations) or commercial actors (for example in business–consumer relations). This vision is increasingly contested as human violations are also committed by individual and corporate parties. Human rights are violated not only by state institutions but also by civil institutions such as the family. In many countries, women's and children's rights are grossly violated within the family. Discrimination, cruelty, violence and censorship often take place within family relations. The place where people should learn first about the respect for others is often the prime locus of violence against others. Human rights are often effectively threatened by people (e.g., by majorities that limit the rights of minorities). Whenever in the world innocent civilians are killed, tortured or raped, this often happens with the silent consent, if not active participation, of other civilians. Also, the poor often violate the human rights of other destitute people. The problem here is that human rights provisions tend to have little effectiveness in spheres outside the realm of the state. This goes back to the liberal origins of human rights protection. It was foreseen by the first human rights drafters (in the 18th century) that citizens needed protection against the state, but protection against fellow citizens was not considered an issue. However, often the perpetrators of human rights abuses are citizens (e.g., in the form of privately owned corporations).

Politics

It is a sobering thought that the post-World War II human rights system was created by a strange assortment of political leaders among which there were Latin American dictators, representatives of authoritarian regimes in Eastern Europe and US politicians who had little desire to be bound by supranational rules. Most likely the political initiators never seriously wanted a universal system of rights for their citizens that would erode their sovereign state powers. The fact that such rights acquired a prominent place on the world agenda is mainly due to the activities of nongovernmental organisations and civil movements. In the late 1940s, it could not be foreseen that civil society would play such a decisive role in the defence of human rights. However, even so, governments have by and large been successful in securing that human rights remain moral standards that were not supported by robust enforcement and remedial measures. It is harmful to the implementation of human rights that the more powerful Western states have repeatedly been hypocritical in their enforcement of human rights standards. Usually human rights violations in so-called client states have been generously overlooked, whereas the readiness to intervene in countries of progressive leaning if they violated human rights has been much greater. Often a double standard has been applied that served geopolitical and economic interests. Cases can be found in the different ways the international community has treated its enemies in Iraq or in former Yugoslavia. Moreover, there is an abundance of cases to demonstrate that many states are willing to trade the defence of human rights for their business interests. The motivation to defend human rights only rarely survives the attractions of commercial contracts. Western attitudes towards the Chinese People's Republic are a case in point. A particularly serious problem in this context is caused by the stakes the five permanent members of the UN Security Council have in the world's arms trade. Almost 90% of the world's weaponry is sold by these five countries. As Garcia-Sayan (1995) rightly observed,

> Weapons on the world market are one of the major sources of corruption of both political and, especially, military institutions. If this issue is not clearly and directly tackled, it is impossible to speak seriously about economic, social, and cultural rights in the Third World.
>
> *(p. 76)*

Despite overwhelming lip-service paid to the respect for human rights, it should be recognised that the desire to seriously implement human rights standards is not universally shared.

Religion

In the major religious movements around the world today, there are certainly strong supporters for the implementation of the international human rights standards. There is a recognition in the different world religions (Christianity, Judaism, Islam, Hinduism and Buddhism) that they share respect for human dignity and basic principles such as tolerance, integrity and equality. Yet the religious support for human rights is not universally shared. It remains in many quarters a contested issue. As a matter of fact, in countries with strong religious presence there is often a great disparity between the theory and the practice of human rights. There is also a long history of gross human rights violations by religious movements. Moreover, today there are traditional religious movements (fundamentalists of various origins) and all kinds of new religious sects that perpetrate – as part of their "sacred mission" – human rights violations as they limit the freedom of conscience of their followers.

In the history of religions, an essential human rights principle such as "freedom of thought, conscience and expression" has always been a contested issue because it fundamentally challenges the institutional hierarchy in religions. Even if religious movements recognise the universality of the human rights principles, their local interpretation may be influenced by religious idiosyncrasies (e.g., ideas on male–female relations) that are difficult to harmonise with these principles. These conflicting interpretations are often defended with references to the Western and imperialist nature of the human rights regime. This is corroborated by the fact that many countries are indeed experiencing a process of cultural colonisation (sometimes referred to as McDonaldization) of which the introduction of human rights is perceived as an important part. This is reinforced by the fact that Western states (and in particular the United States) have so often practiced human rights imperialism in the pursuit of their foreign policy. Against this, the supporters of human rights in religious movements will propose that conflicting interpretations of human rights principles can be resolved by rethinking the religious doctrines. However, this may not be so easy because there are real differences between religious and secular conceptions on the notion of "rights". The disparity between the secular conception that rights are derived from inherent human dignity is not so easily reconciled with the theocentric position that rights are the gift of God. In the latter view, rights are obtained on the basis of the fulfilment of obligations towards the Divine Will. In line with this, it should also be recognised that in most world religions the dominant discourse is about duties and not about rights.

In the religious world of the Islam, a complex question is also whether Islamic conformity with human rights principles should also imply that Shari'a should be in conformity with human rights standards. Shari'a comprises "the laws derived from the Qu'ran, the Sunnah, the Hadith and decisions of Muhammed, Ijma' – the consensus of opinion of the Ulama (Judges) and Ijtihad – the counsel of judges on a particular case" (Traer, 1991, p. 115). If conformity of national jurisdiction with Shari'a is demanded, as the fundamentalist theologians certainly would prefer, there is an insurmountable problem. Although the Qu'ran may contain paragraphs that support religious liberty, this is not the case in Shari'a and has often not been the political practice in Muslim countries where the state has the responsibility to enforce the Shari'a. Shari'a fundamentally rejects such basic human rights principles as non-discrimination and equality: "it is impossible for Shari'a to acknowledge any set of rights to which all human beings are entitled by virtue of their humanity, without distinction on grounds of religion or gender" (An-Na'im et al., 1995, p. 238).

Economics: Globalisation

The effects of the processes of economic globalisation on the defence of human rights are not homogeneous. In different societies and in different strata of the same society, these effects are different. Globalisation processes may both promote and threaten human rights. Global network technologies strengthen free speech but also disseminate hate speech. At the core of economic globalisation stands a societal model in which economic and contractual relations determine the nature of social relations. In the modern contract society, human rights are subsumed under economic rationales, and its key actors are driven primarily by self-centred interests. This clashes with human rights standards that are inspired by compassion with the interests of others.

It is a peculiar development that in current economic globalisation there is a strong drive towards deregulation and a minimal role for the state, whereas in the 19th and 20th centuries societies learned that deregulated free markets spell enormous social disaster. As Ghai (1999) argued "few states, even the colonial, have found it possible or expedient to let markets unfold in the fullness of their logic, because the consequences of free markets threaten social peace and stability". (p. 245) Government had to intervene to keep the social costs of free markets under control. Modern markets, despite all the claims to freedom, are dependent on the coercive power of national states. This power benefits some people more than others. If, on the national level, free markets pose serious threats to social stability, people's welfare and natural resources, it is difficult to see why anyone would expect that the project of a global free market would not face instability, poverty and resource depletion. A close reading of current statements and reflections on economic globalisation does not reveal any serious argument to support the thesis that global autonomous markets would cause any less disaster than would national autonomous markets.

As the role of the market becomes more dominant in modern societies, the outcome is in general more access to better educational and health services for few people and a deterioration of welfare for most people. The marketisation of societies clashes fundamentally with the concept of human rights on the issue of equality. Whereas equality is a core standard in international human rights, the modern market does not foster equality.

Conflicting Human Rights

The implementation of human rights is often problematic as a result of conflicts among human rights, conflicts between human rights and significant societal interests or conflicts between human rights and cultural values.

Rights Versus Rights

A classical case is the situation in which the human right to the protection of privacy (Article 12 of the UDHR) conflicts with the human right to freedom of expression (Article 19 of the UDHR) or situations in which the free speech standard clashes with the prohibition to discriminate. This is complicated because there is no hierarchy of rights that can provide a definitive arbitration. A crucial characteristic of the human rights regime is the indivisibility of its constituent rights. In 1993, the UN World Conference on Human Rights (at Vienna) emphasised this by stating, "All human rights are universal, indivisible and interdependent and interrelated". In the conflict among human rights, one can only neglect one category of rights at the expense of other rights. In reality, however, situations that represent irresolvable dilemmas occur infrequently. In most situations, dilemmas can be resolved when the pertinent elements of a confrontation are adequately analysed. The analysis often shows that one of the claims is ill-founded. Although rights can be considered of equal significance, the grounds on which their realisation is claimed may be of a different order. It may well be that the claim to the protection of privacy is grounded on a limited private interest, whereas the claim to free speech is based on a broad public interest. If the parties involved fail to resolve this conflict through the social dialogue, courts of law will usually come to acceptable judgments.

Rights Versus Significant Interests

This conflict has become prominent after the events of September 11, 2001. In the aftermath of the attacks in the United States, human rights (such as the protection of privacy, free speech, due process of law) across the world have been severely limited on grounds of national security and the war against terrorism. As Ronald Dworkin (2002) wrote in an essay for the *New York Review of Books*,

> What has al-Qaeda done to our Constitution, and to our national standards of fairness and decency? Since September 11, the government has enacted legislation, adopted policies, and threatened procedures that are not consistent with our established laws and values and would have been unthinkable before.
>
> *(p. 44)*

After September 11, the international agreement to cooperate against terrorism has shifted to the language of "war on terrorism". For human rights, this is problematic because the emphasis in many states came to be on security and order, and many national experiences have demonstrated that this tends to go together with limits to the enjoyment of basic rights. The core difficulty is this: because no human right – however fundamental – can be absolute, there is always the possibility that significant national or personal interests demand qualification of basic rights.

However, because this qualification may undermine human rights to unacceptable levels, each conflict between rights and interests needs to be judged in light of the following four criteria.

- **Proportionality:** is the restriction of a right proportional to the protection of the proposed aim? In other words, is there a pressing social need for the restriction?
- **Subsidiarity:** is there no alternative measure to achieve the proposed aim?
- **Effectiveness:** is there evidence that the proposed restriction will indeed achieve the proposed aim?
- **Duration:** is the restriction only of a temporary duration?

Rights Versus Cultural Values

Under this heading, one finds conflicts between the right to physical integrity and the cultural practice of female genital mutilation, between the right to freedom of religion and culture-specific religious rulings (like fatwas) or between the right to be protected against discrimination and culture-based rejections of homosexuality. In such conflicts, it should always be questioned whose cultural values are at stake. What is presented as the cultural preferences of whole communities often only reflects the bias and interest of a cultural elite. Moreover, it should be realised that cultures are human constructs and, as such, are changeable and not sacrosanct.

More often than not, the cultural argument is based on a selective interpretation of a culture's sources (e.g., its sacred scriptures), and a different reading of these sources may not conflict with human rights standards. Although many rights versus culture conflicts can probably be resolved in a serious dialogue among those concerned, it should not be ignored that there may indeed be situations in which the standards of international human rights law and those cherished by cultural communities clash in non-negotiable ways.

The Justiciability and Universality of Human Rights

An important question for the realisation of human rights is their justiciability. This means that courts of law assist in the protection of human rights. Can national litigation processes help the enforcement of international rights? An crucial condition for this would be that states bind themselves to these rights through UN bodies or adopt these rights as part of their domestic legislation. There is disagreement in the literature on the issue whether courts of law should dictate political choice in matters of human rights. There also is a general agreement that law courts could demand from political policy-makers that they in cases concerning the realisation of human rights publicly justify their choices. Courts of law could also give a voice to those who would otherwise be excluded from the public debate.

In the different human rights instruments we find striking similarities on essential principles such as equality, security and freedom. Actually, these similarities are not so surprising even if we accept the reality of the world's cultural diversity, because there are remarkably few people that publicly support racism, slavery or genocide. If one accepts that moral standards are culturally relative, this does not imply that there cannot be universal moral standards. When people differ about the value of certain customs and practices, they may very well share the same basic moral premises. The ways in which cultural communities approach the treatment of the deceased, male–female relations or the education of children may be totally different. Yet, they may be based on the same moral principles. Burying, cremating, embalming or eating the dead may all be inspired by the same respect for those who passed away.

Postmodernists object to universal moral principles or truths and favour the tolerance of pluralism. However, how can one hope to achieve tolerance without shared normative principles? Why should we be tolerant? Does tolerance of plural truths not imply the respect for the universal moral principle of the tolerance of diversity? The postmodern relativists claim that there can be no universal claims. It remains unclear, though, how they substantiate this claim. It would seem reasonable to expect that they demonstrate empirically that no universal norms exist.

The issue is not whether all or most moral norms are universally accepted but whether there are any shared principles at all. And, indeed, it is difficult to ignore that there is a limited set of basic norms that most people across time and space share! One of the problems with a relativist position is that there is little hope for justification outside the boundaries of a specific situation. Thus moral relativism may ultimately lead to moral indifference for events beyond the confines of a local scheme of values. Against this, the universalist position accepts that there are values that transcend local boundaries and that these are applicable to all. The universalist refuses to abandon the world and people's common future to moral indifference.

Most essential for the universal significance of human rights standards is the observation that they constitute the only global moral framework that the international community has at present. This was – after much discussion – clearly confirmed by the 1993 UN World Conference on Human Rights in Vienna. This Conference stated in its unanimously adopted declaration,

> The World Conference on Human Rights reaffirms the solemn commitment of all States to fulfil their obligations to promote universal respect for, and observance and protection of, all human rights and fundamental freedoms for all in accordance with the Charter of the United Nations, other instruments relating to human rights, and international law. The universal nature of these rights and freedoms is beyond question.

Although this was an important step, the recognition of universal validity did not resolve the question of the admissible variety of cultural interpretations. Universal validity does not mean that all local forms of implementation are similar. A variety of cultural interpretations remains possible. This has provoked the question of to what degree local cultural interpretations can be accepted. There is increasing support for the view that culturally determined interpretations reach a borderline when they violate the core principles of human rights law. Moreover, this view holds that the admissibility of the interpretation should be judged by the international community and not by the implementing party. Given the world's diversity of cultures and the fact that human rights will only be taken seriously if they are seen as culturally legitimate, the reference in the 1993 Vienna declaration to the need of cultural interpretations makes sense.

However, questions remain. What universality is left once cultural interpretations are fundamentally in conflict? For example, in the case of religions that only accept the authority of their sacred texts and authorised interpretations of such texts, if human rights texts prevail over religious texts or the other way around, there may be a non-negotiable conflict.

Another problem with the issue of cultural interpretation is posed by the flawed assumption of homogeneous cultures that totally bypasses the existing internal diversity in cultural communities. There are always in all cultures traditionalists versus modernists, for example. The West is often portrayed as a homogeneous cultural entity! But is it? Does the West exist? If so, since when? Is it a reality or merely an ideological by-product of the cold war? In the early stages of the UN, only 13 out of 51 member states perceived of themselves as Western. Only 6 of the 18 members on the Human Rights Commission considered themselves Western. Interestingly, the Chinese were in favour of non-discrimination and equal rights provisions in the UDHR, whereas the United States and the United Kingdom opposed these. Actually, at the time of the League of Nations, Japan wanted to ban racism but lost to the United States, the United Kingdom and France. A troublesome assumption is also the construction of totally distinct value systems between the East and West (e.g., in the idea of a juxtaposition of an Asian collectivism versus a Western individualism). It could be, however, that the West turns out to be less individualistic than some Asian political elites propose. There is more collective social security in the West than in many Asian countries. The common good is important in many Western countries. Actually, taxation for the common good is common in the West. One often finds the accusation that Western values lead to crime and drug abuse. It would also be good to reflect on Asian values and the levels of pollution in Asian cities, the widespread occurrence of AIDS and booming criminality. Moreover, it may be that so-called individual rights like the right to free speech serve collective purposes like democracy and that the right to free association represents a claim for community and social solidarity. It is often said that the human rights tradition is exclusively focused on individual rights. It is certainly true that human rights are to an important extent articulated in the language of a Western individualistic liberal tradition. However, this does not hinder the provision of collective rights, such as the rights of minorities. In the evolution of human rights, the link between individual and collective rights has become stronger. Moreover, individual rights are always tied to the rights of other members of the community and the community at large.

As Article 29 of the Universal Declaration of Human Rights provides: "everyone has duties to the community in which alone the free and full development of his personality is possible". The real controversy, however, is not between individual versus collective rights but is about whether people are entitled to being treated decently by their state, society, tribe, clan, family and partners. Can this entitlement be realised universally so that no one is excluded?

Abdul Aziz Said (1998) wrote, "Human rights may be difficult to define but impossible to ignore". (p. xi) It is indeed true that in the early 21st century human rights have become a reality, but so have their worldwide violation. As nationalism and anti-multi-lateralism are on the rise worldwide, universality is threatened by racism, xenophobia and state legislations designed to guarantee the fundamental rights of the citizens of their countries. The access to human rights for non-citizens is challenged by the anchoring of human rights in the nation-state and citizenship and the boundedness of human rights to the exclusionary structures of liberal democracy. The failures of the global governance system to deal with people's concerns about inequality, poverty, exploitation, extraction, climate and war led to the rapid growth of extreme right-wing parties with totalitarian features and strong nationalist sentiments. Populist movements pit the "true" people against the enemies and offer simple solutions for complex problems. They pose a threat to multilateral institutions and international cooperation in the field of health. Nationalist populism undermines the protection of global human rights.

Enforcement: The United Nations

The key problem in human rights enforcement is the absence of a functioning global regulatory infrastructure to implement the universal moral aspirations human rights embody. To create such an infrastructure in the 21st century, we would have to begin with the transformation of the only global forum for human rights, which is the UN. Although the preamble of its Charter (1945) announces "we the peoples of the United Nations", the organisation never became an association of nations. The UN became an association of states. And states and nations are very different entities even though the odd notion of the "nation-state" suggests otherwise. A state is an administrative unit with a monopoly on the use of force whereas a nation refers to people sharing a common heritage and a common cultural understanding. Real nations are the Inuit, the Maori, the Masaai, the Australian aboriginals or the Zapotec Indians. An association of states is inherently incapable of creating global politics "as if people mattered". States are by and large self-centred and practice only a limited form of altruism. They tend more towards competition than towards cooperation. Their interests are primarily provincial and not global. States are often unreliable as they frequently are masters in deception and propaganda. States are minimally interested in diversity. They would like their polities to be homogeneous with one language, one culture and a single moral framework. Many states have little interest in change. There may be revolutions, but once enough people have been killed everything goes back to "business as usual". From Darwinian biology we know that altruism, cooperation, diversity and change are essential conditions for the survival of a species. It seems fair to assume that the same goes for institutions. From this perspective the UN is very unfit to manage global affairs in a sustainable way. The failure of the 15-member UN Security Council to uphold its mandate of maintaining international peace and security when in early 2022 Russia invaded Ukraine in violation of the UN Charter demonstrated its irrelevance. The sentinel of global peace and security has outlived its usefulness when, in spite of overwhelming opposition of members of the UN General Assembly, an aggressive war cannot be avoided. The UN organisation urgently needs transformation from a global association that presents statal interests towards a global people's association that defends people's interests. This institution would need to be embedded in a social and international order in which human rights can be fully realised.

Concluding Remarks

The international community has – in response to the gross violence of the Second World War – designed a normative framework that sets standards for the behaviour of institutions and individuals. Its basis is the UDHR from which declarations, resolutions and treaties did originate that require realisation in concrete situations such as the practice of health care on a global scale. Even after many decades, this realisation has not yet been achieved. This should inspire us to "strive by teaching and education to promote respect for these rights and freedoms and by progressive measures, national and international, to secure their universal and effective recognition and observance" (UN,1948).

Questions for Discussion

- Discuss with friends, family or colleagues concrete examples of unequal treatment and/or acts of humiliation that you have witnessed.
- As the planet is a universe that encompasses all sentient beings – among which are humans – the question arises whether the term "human" rights is not too anthropocentric. Does it not suggest that the planet is a "humans only" affair? How can we extend the principles of dignity, equality, freedom and security to all life on planet Earth?
- There is also an issue with the concept of "rights". Since states give rights and can take them away, do rights not imply a situation of dependency? Right is a very legalistic concept, and the question is how well it works for non-human entities such as rivers and mountains. Many rights-bearers (also humans, like people with dementia) cannot stand up for themselves and they are dependent for the protection of their rights upon the moral behaviour of others. As the year 2023 celebrates the 75th anniversary of the Universal Declaration of Human Rights, this could be an opportune time to adopt a Universal Declaration of Human Responsibilities, as was proposed in 1997, which would complement the Human Rights Declaration and strengthen it. Discuss how a declaration of human responsibilities would treat health and health care.
- Discuss with friends, family or colleagues whether "informed consent" is a realistic demand under all conditions.
- Discuss with friends, family or colleagues whether governmental measures in your country during the COVID-19 pandemic met these criteria.
- Discuss with friends, family or colleagues how proposals for mandatory vaccination against coronavirus (SARS-CoV-2) relate to the principle of human autonomy.
- Discuss with friends, family or colleagues how you – as judge in a court of law – would judge in a conflict between the protection of public health and the protection of basic civil rights such as the right to free movement.

References

An-Na'im, A. A., Groot, J. D., Jansen, H., & Vroom, H. M. (Eds.). (1995). *Human rights and religious values*. William B. Eerdmans Publishing.

Dworkin, R. (2002). The threat to patriotism. *The New York Review of Books*, XLIX(3), 44–50.

Garcia-Sayan, D. (1995). New path for economic, social and cultural rights. *The Review: International Commission of Jurists*, 55, 75–80.

Ghai, Y. (1999). Rights, social justice and globalization in East Asia. In J. R. Bauer & D. A. Bell (Eds.), *The East Asian challenge for human rights* (pp. 241–263). Cambridge University Press.

Jongman, J. J., & Schmidt, A. P. (1994). *Monitoring human rights*. PIOOM.

Partsch, K. J. (1981). Freedom of expression and conscience, and political freedom. In L. Henkin (Ed.), *The international bill of rights* (pp. 209–245). Hampton Press.

Said, A. A. (Ed.). (1998). *Human rights in world order*. Praeger.

Traer, R. (1991). *Faith in human rights*. Georgetown University Press.

UN. (1945). *Charter of the United Nations.* https://www.un.org/en/charter-united-nations/

UN. (1948). *Universal Declaration of Human Rights.* https://www.un.org/en/about-us/universal-declaration-of-human-rights

UN Committee on Economic, Social and Cultural Rights. (1993). *Report on the seventh session, 23 November–11 December 1992 (E/1993/22).* United Nations.

For Further Reading

Baehr, P. (1999). *Human rights: Universality in practice.* Palgrave Macmillan.

Benhabib, S. (2011). *Dignity in adversity: Human rights in troubled times.* Polity Press.

Dundes Renteln, A. (1990). *International human rights: Universalism versus relativism.* Sage.

Ishay, N. (2004). *The history of human rights.* The University of California Press.

Jacobson, M., & Bruhn, O. (2000). *Human rights and Asian values.* Curzon Press.

Nickel, J. W. (1987). *Making sense of human rights.* The University of California Press.

Othman, N. (1999). Grounding human rights arguments in non-Western culture. In J. R. Bauer & D. A. Bell (Eds.), *The East Asian challenge for human rights* (pp. 169–192). Cambridge University Press.

Pogge, T. (2002). *World poverty and human rights.* Polity Press.

Posner, E. A. (2014). *The twilight of human rights law.* Oxford University Press.

Steiner, H. J., & Alston, P. (2000). *International human rights in context.* Oxford University Press.

Woodiwiss, A. (2005). *Human rights.* Routledge.

CHAPTER 2

An Introduction to Global Health

Abdul K. Azad and Dirk R. Essink

Introduction

In this second chapter, we begin by offering a brief historical account of global health. This account aims to define global health, trace its development and highlight its foundation in human rights. Equally important, this historical perspective underscores the significant challenges that persist in global health today, many of which are deeply rooted in its past. For instance, global health funding agencies and research institutions are still predominantly based in the Global North, and global health knowledge production and implementation often fail to incorporate local knowledge.

While the chapter addresses the colonial roots of contemporary global health practices, it is important to note that the chapter itself starts from a Eurocentric perspective. This narrative also reveals the complexities of distinguishing global health practice from public health. The chapter refrains from providing an exhaustive overview of various global health topics, such as maternal health and malnutrition. For further reading, please refer to the list at the end of the chapter.

Learning Objectives

After studying this chapter you will be able to:

- Understand the origin and scope of global health
- Understand how the human rights and global health discourse are intertwined
- Understand social determinants of health and how they relate to equity
- Understand that despite intertwinement there are large disparities in health outcomes and power differences between actors from the Global North and South
- Understand what is meant by epistemic (in)justice and decolonising global health

DOI: 10.4324/9781003408765-4

A Short History of Global Health

Imperialism and Tropical Medicine

During the age of "exploration, colonisation and exploitation", European powers seized control of vast geographical areas, exploiting both the land and its people. This period also saw the unintended introduction of new diseases to Indigenous populations. Diseases such as smallpox, measles and influenza, which were common in Europe, had devastating effects on communities with no prior exposure or immunity, leading to widespread epidemics and significant population declines. In the Americas, Indigenous communities experienced catastrophic depopulation, with estimates of declines ranging from 75% to 95% (Livi-Bacci, 2006). From this dark chapter in history, the field of global health began to emerge.

During that time, global health was often referred to as "colonial", "missionary" or "military" medicine and later more formally as "tropical medicine". While fields like epidemiology, public health and surgery were also deployed within colonial settings, tropical medicine specifically aimed to support and expand colonisation efforts. Its primary focus was on addressing diseases that affected settlers, merchants and the military. Reflecting the prevailing racist and class ideologies, the best health care was reserved for European colonisers, with limited health care provided to those deemed useful to them. Similarly to modern global health, tropical medicine emphasised research. Many European global health institutes still bear names that reflect this legacy, such as the Institute of Tropical Medicine and Hygiene in London, the Royal Tropical Institute in Amsterdam and the Prince Leopold Institute of Tropical Medicine in Antwerp. In the postcolonial era, these institutions have continued to thrive, often continuing the legacy of colonialism (Affun-Adegbulu et al., 2023). During the same period, the All India Institute of Hygiene and Public Health (AIIHPH) was established in Kolkata, India. However, its output and prestige rank poorly compared to its European counterparts.

A substantial part of the research at the time drew from existing Indigenous knowledge systems which were later co-opted by colonisers. For example, the use of quinine from the bark of the cinchona tree to treat malaria was practiced by Indigenous populations in South America long before it was documented by Jesuit missionaries in the 16th century. The French explorer and scientist Charles Marie de La Condamine was the first to publish how to use it effectively, and by the 1820s quinine had been isolated and refined. Until the 1940s, it remained the preferred treatment for malaria, and it was only in 2006 that the WHO ceased recommending its use due to the availability of alternatives with fewer side effects. Quinine was rapidly adopted to protect colonisers, who had little natural immunity, thereby becoming a powerful tool of imperialism. It was also used in Europe, where malaria was still endemic.

Tropical medicine also contributed to understanding the link between diet and disease. Nobel Prize winner Christiaan Eijkman, sent as an army doctor to the Dutch East Indies, was struck by the number of soldiers incapacitated by beriberi. Contrary to the prevailing belief that beriberi was infectious, he demonstrated that it was caused by a vitamin B1 deficiency, making him one of the first to highlight the importance of vitamins in our diets.

The examples of quinine and beriberi demonstrate that while tropical medicine did contribute to scientific advancement, its primary motivation was to support colonial oppression. Other aspects of colonial and tropical medicine were far more gruesome. Experimentation on enslaved persons was common; for example, enslaved people were used to study the reproductive system to increase the "production of slaves". Pseudo-medical experiments were conducted to assert white superiority, such as craniometry (measuring skull size) to justify racial hierarchies and the theory of "exotic syphilis", which falsely claimed that most Arabs suffered from hereditary syphilis, rendering them feeble and less intelligent (Amster, 2016). These studies were profoundly unethical, scientifically baseless and constituted acts of torture.

The Public Health Movement

In the 19th and early 20th century, welfare programs expanded, including in colonies. Public health movements emerged, advocating for better sanitation, housing and working conditions, particularly to combat infectious diseases and high fertility rates in rapidly growing urban centres. The role of science and evidence-informed decision-making based on epidemiological data gained prominence following John Snows' investigation of Cholera epidemics in London (Vinten-Johansen, 2003). The public acceptance of "germ-theory", spurred by the (bio-)medical innovations of Louis Pasteur, Robert Koch, Ian Flemming and members of the community of tropical medicine, further advanced public health. They introduced biomedical interventions such as vaccines and antibiotics to the largely preventive public health movement (Gaynes, 2023). This integration of epidemiological and biomedical research remains the backbone of global health today.

Although the emergence of the public health movement showed the first signs of striving for more equitable health outcomes, injustices remained pervasive. This initial public health movement lacked the moral underpinnings of social justice that characterise it today. At that time, public health practices were often instrumental in attaining power and wealth. For instance, in Germany, Chancellor Otto von Bismarck initiated a national health insurance plan for workers and their families to counter the rising popularity of socialist parties and ensure a healthy workforce and military (Tulchinsky, 2018). Humiliation, discrimination, coercion and inequalities were rampant both in in the "colonised world" as well as within imperialist countries. As Anna Greenwood (2022) states,

> even after World War 1 when colonial medical provision expanded to rural areas – culminating in the Colonial Development and Welfare Acts of the 1940s – the methods deployed by colonial doctors continued to be racist and inequitable. Medical treatments were often enforced, people were moved with little explanation away from their families and homes, and local people who had infectious diseases were sometimes instructed to carry health passports and had differential access to health facilities. Indigenous medical beliefs were derided as superstitious and non-efficacious with little cultural sensitivity, and local people were sometimes coercively and often unwillingly involved in medical research projects.
>
> *(p. 727)*

Human Rights and International Health

After World War II, it all changed, at least on paper. Health became a core ambition of the newly established UN and its "ministry of health", the World Health Organisation

(WHO). The WHO was tasked with operationalising human rights in public health, primarily focusing on low- and middle-income settings. At that time, the WHO introduced its ground-breaking definition of health: "health is a state of complete physical, mental and social well-being and not merely the absence of disease or infirmity". This was revolutionary at the time, as it expanded the concept of health beyond the mere absence of disease to include social and mental well-being. Despite facing criticism over the years, this definition remains influential more than 65 years later.

This period also marked the increasing intertwining of global health and human rights, becoming known as international health. The right to health encompasses various socio-economic factors that create conditions for a healthy life. These fundamental health determinants include food and nutrition, housing, access to safe and potable water, adequate sanitation, safe and healthy working conditions and a healthy environment. Within global health, these factors are referred to as the social determinants of health (SDH), arguably the most important framework in global health research and practice (see Textbox 2.1). For more information on the "right to health", see Chapter 3 of this book. Parallel to these rights movements, the welfare state expanded in most high-income countries, making health care increasingly universally accessible and improving health outcomes.

However, the inequalities between different parts of the globe grew rapidly, even though formal colonisation had ended (for examples, see later discussion). Although most countries, to varying degrees, acknowledge the right to health, the availability, accessibility, acceptability and quality of health care in many low- and middle-income countries (LMICs) lagged far behind. For example, since 1900, the global average life expectancy has more than doubled and is now above 70 years. Yet the life expectancy gap between high- and low-income countries is a staggering 18 years, not accounting for life lost due to disability. The international health response to these challenges focused on applying public health principles to address issues such as infectious diseases, malnutrition, hygiene, sanitation and maternal and child health, issues that predominantly affect LMIC (Brown et al., 2006; Koplan et al., 2009). The period of international health also saw the emergence of many small-scale participatory projects, and participatory action research methodology gained increasing recognition within the field. However, participation was often limited to small communal settings, with actual decision-making often determined by donors.

Textbox 2.1
The Social Determinants of Health (SDH)

The SDH are the non-medical factors that impact health outcomes. They encompass the conditions in which individuals are born, grow, work, live and age, as well as the broader array of influences shaping daily life like income and social protection; education; unemployment and job insecurity; working life conditions; food insecurity; housing; basic amenities and the environment; early childhood development; social inclusion and non-discrimination; structural conflict; and access to affordable health services of decent quality.

The SDH significantly impact health inequities, which refer to the unjust and preventable disparities in health status observed within and among nations. The WHO states that the social determinants influence health outcomes more than health care services or individual lifestyle choices and that the social determinants account for 30–55% of health outcomes. Furthermore, estimates reveal that sectors beyond health care make a greater contribution to population health outcomes compared to the health care sector. Regardless of a country's income level, health outcomes typically follow a social gradient: individuals in lower socio-economic positions tend to experience poorer health.

Acknowledging the influence of SDH is crucial for achieving equity in health care. This involves the redistribution of resources for health between persons and communities to ensure universal health coverage (UHC).

Global Health

In the latter half of the 20th century and into the 21st century, it became increasingly apparent that health challenges are not confined by national borders or limited to LMICs. Globalisation accelerated the movement of people, goods, information and culture, allowing both communicable and non-communicable diseases and their determinants to transcend geopolitical boundaries The term "global health" reflects this reality and emphasises the need for collaboration and cross-border solutions. For example, the HIV/AIDS epidemic, along with the stigma associated with it, affected people across the globe. Discriminatory and coercive practices such as compulsory testing, named reporting, travel restrictions and isolation or quarantine were counterproductive, exacerbating stigma and impeding effective responses. A global movement was needed to challenge conservative and corporate power and ensure access to medicine, support and prevention. Similarly, the outbreak of SARS led to the revision of the International Health Regulations (IHR) (2005), emphasising the necessity of cross-border collaboration. The Framework Convention on Tobacco Control (2003) was another example of a transnational, multistakeholder agreement effort to combat risk factors. These examples illustrate the need for global and interdisciplinary cooperation between stakeholders from science and society to address these challenges. This includes professionals from fields such as medicine, public health, economics, sociology, anthropology, ethics and environmental science.

The future of global health is likely to see more integration with the current field of planetary health, a field that focuses on understanding the interconnections between human health and the health of the planet's natural systems. It recognises that human health is deeply interconnected with the health of the environment, including ecosystems, biodiversity, climate systems and other planetary processes.

Defining Global Health

The evolution of global health reveals its origins in colonial and tropical medicine. While global health has largely maintained a focus on how diseases, risk factors and responses vary across geographical areas, it recognises that these issues are not confined to specific locations, with research remaining a central focus. The public health movement laid the groundwork for addressing population health and health care equity, driven by the moral conviction of the right to health. This shift led the international health community to increasingly prioritise improving health care in the Global South. Concurrently, health and disease began to be understood within the framework of social determinants of health (SDH).

In the past two decades, the term "international health" has been replaced with "global health". According to Koplan et al. (2009, p. 1995), global health is defined as

> an area for study, research, and practice that places a priority on improving health and achieving equity in health for all people worldwide. Global health emphasises transnational health issues, determinants, and solutions; involves many disciplines within and beyond the health sciences and promotes interdisciplinary collaboration; and is a synthesis of population-based prevention with individual-level clinical care.

Dissecting this definition, we first have to establish that global health is normative; it strives to "achieve equity in health outcomes" (see Textbox 2.1 and Salm et al., 2021). This implies that global health has a focus on those most affected by worse health outcomes, increasingly taking an intersectional lens (Kapilashrami & Hankivsky, 2018; also see Chapter 5). For example, how can we achieve equity in health outcomes for rural, poor women from ethnic minorities in a low-income setting? However, unlike with international health, global health also focuses on people that are "vulnerable" in high-income settings. Critically, "global" goes beyond LMIC and encompasses health concerns that affect numerous countries or are influenced by transnational factors like climate change, urbanisation or shared solutions such as polio eradication. While the historical focal topics like maternal and child health and infectious diseases (e.g., Dengue, Influenza A (H5N1) and HIV) clearly fall within the global health domain, global health also encompasses broader issues such as tobacco control, micronutrient deficiencies, obesity, injury prevention, migrant-worker health and the migration of health workers. The term "global" in global health signifies the breadth of problems addressed, not just their geographical location. Unlike the more restrictive focus of international health, global health can examine domestic health disparities in addition to cross-border issues and health issues of "vulnerable" people in high-income settings. The third aspect is specific inclusion of personal medicine in addition to population health. Partly driven by the increasing burden of chronic diseases, the need for universal coverage of high-quality health services is critical. Under the heading of health system strengthening, in the past decades the global health community has emphasised that strong health systems are required to implement disease-specific approaches. This goes beyond the traditional scope of public health, extending to the training and distribution of the health care workforce in ways that go beyond requirements for public health initiatives. Koplan et al. (2009) and Salm et al. (2021) underline that global health requires interdisciplinary, multisectoral and culturally sensitive approaches for reducing health disparities that transcend national borders.

Textbox 2.2
Equity

Equity entails eliminating unjust, preventable or correctable variances among social, economic, demographic or geographic groups, as well as other dimensions of inequality such as sex, gender, ethnicity, disability or sexual orientation. Health, a fundamental human entitlement, is realised when all individuals can reach their maximum potential for health and well-being.

To explain equity, educators often turn to the following picture. The picture shows three persons of varying height who (attempt to) watch a baseball match. The pitch is surrounded by a fence and all three stand on a crate. The first two persons can see over the fence while the third, while standing on one crate, cannot. The picture portrays equality; everyone has one crate, but the outcome is unequal, only two can watch the match. In the second picture, the tallest person has no crate and the smallest person has two. The situation is unequal in its division of crates but equal in its outcome – everybody can watch over the fence. The latter, equality of outcome, is called equity. A similar graphic exists about three people of different height trying to pick an apple from an applet tree. First, the smallest person cannot reach the apple. After redistributing the crates, all can pick an apple.

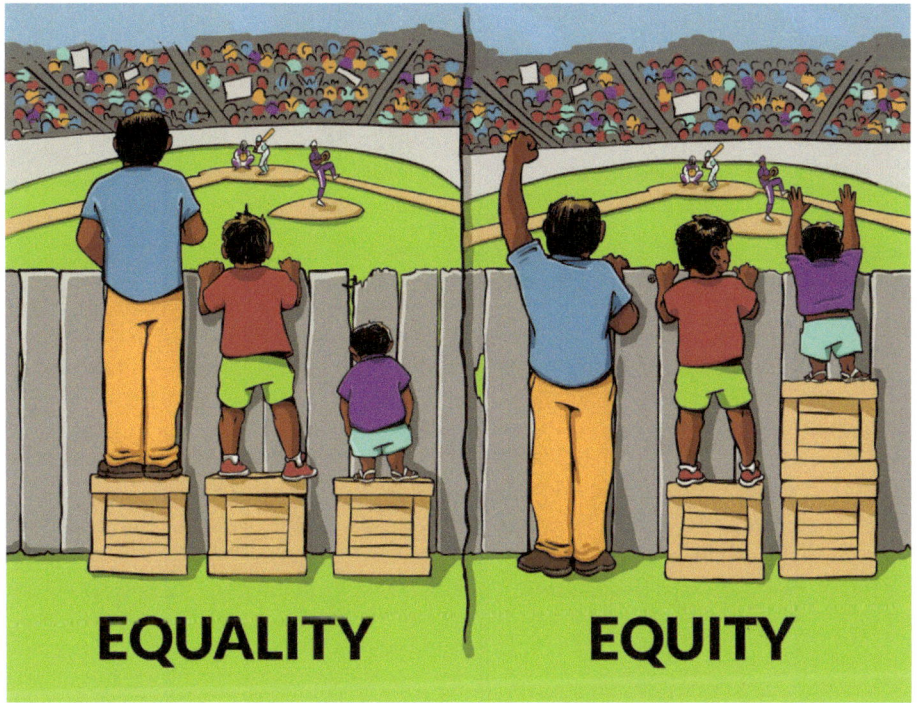

Figure 2.1 Equality and Equity (Image credit: Interaction Institute for Social Change | Artist: Angus Maguire)

Providing the crate may have led to equality of outcome, but if achieving equity is merely about offering additional resources to marginalised groups – such as reducing health care premiums for the less privileged or providing food allowances to marginalised communities, as symbolised by the crates – we are not truly tackling the root causes of the issue. In fact, such measures might inadvertently disempower those in need, as they become passive recipients rather than active participants in solving their own challenges.

In the baseball match scenario, the fence represents the structural problem. Sometimes, the wooden fence is replaced by a see-through fence or by removing it altogether, which is labelled as "justice" or "liberation". In case of the apple tree, there is no barrier that can be changed but it is the apple tree itself which is too tall and needs to be changed – such as a shorter trunk or lower-hanging branches. Alternatively, the apple tree might illustrate inherent differences between individuals – such as height – that cannot be easily changed. A fully equitable society remains a goal worth striving for, though it may be an unattainable goal. Having said that, it is important to recognise that both scenarios are problematic, as they perpetuate the notion that being smaller or having differences is something that needs compensation.

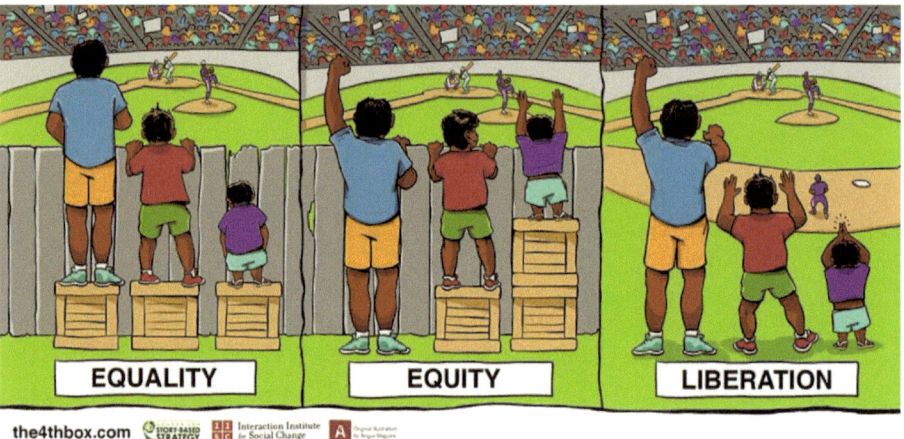

Figure 2.2 Equality, Equity and Liberation Equality and Equity (Image credit: a collaboration between Center for Story-based Strategy and Interaction Institute for Social Change)

Well, either way, both the baseball match and the apple tree illustrations illustrate the concept of equality of outcome and how equity differs from equality. They also support reflection on how social systems reproduce inequalities. Therefore, we should strive for what we call equity-specific interventions; strategies designed to address immediate and acute inequities. Examples include providing free or low-cost health care to those who cannot afford it or offering additional support to children with disabilities to facilitate their participation in sports.

However, societies require equity-sensitive interventions – those that address the underlying social structures creating inequities: such as the fence you cannot see through or the apple tree that is too tall. Simply replacing these structures is often not the ideal solution. For instance, while the fence may be oppressive to some, it also serves a protective function, ensuring safety during the match. Equity-sensitive interventions require just transformations that consider the social goals of these structures. For the fence, this might mean redesigning it to be transparent while still maintaining safety. In the case of the apple tree, solutions are less straightforward due to the complexity of the issue. Equity-sensitive transformations are inherently complex and necessitate changes across multiple levels of social systems. In Chapter 13 of this book, we explore a scenario-based approach to support critical thinking about equitable solutions.

Arguably the most important global effort to improve global health is embedded within the 17 UN Sustainable Development Goals (SDGs). SDG3 specifically addresses health and well-being, whereas other SDGs focus on important determinants of health. For example, SDG 1 aims to reduce poverty, and SDG 2 aims to improve food security. Other SDG goals emphasise access to education, (gender) equality, economic opportunities and environmental goals. See Textbox 2.3 for the targets for 2030 of SDG3. However, most of the targets of SDG 3 (and others) are off track for meeting the 2030 goals. For example, the 2023 maternal death ratio of "223/100,000 live births" still exceeds the 2030 target of 70 maternal deaths per 100,000 live births (WHO). Also, the SDGs are increasingly seen as driven by the "Global North", overemphasising long-term environmental goals, whereas the Global South's direct needs – such as improved well-being, ending poverty, improving food security and access to energy – may compromise the environmental goals (Vogt, 2022).

Textbox 2.3
SDG3 to "Ensure Healthy Lives and Promote Well-being for All at All Ages"

- Target 3.1: by 2030, reduce the global maternal mortality ratio to less than 70 per 100,000 live births.
- Target 3.2: by 2030, end preventable deaths of new-borns and children under 5 years of age, with all countries aiming to reduce neonatal mortality to at least as low as 12 per 1,000 live births and under-5 mortality to at least as low as 25 per 1,000 live births.
- Target 3.3: by 2030, end the epidemics of AIDS, tuberculosis, malaria and neglected tropical diseases and combat hepatitis, water-borne diseases and other communicable diseases.
- Target 3.4: by 2030, reduce by one third premature mortality from non-communicable diseases through prevention and treatment and promote mental health and well-being.
- Target 3.5: strengthen the prevention and treatment of substance abuse, including narcotic drug abuse and harmful use of alcohol.
- Target 3.6: by 2030, halve the number of global deaths and injuries from road traffic accidents.
- Target 3.7: by 2030, ensure universal access to sexual and reproductive health care services, including for family planning, information and education and the integration of reproductive health into national strategies and programs.
- Target 3.8: achieve universal health coverage, including financial risk protection, access to quality essential health care services and access to safe, effective, quality and affordable essential medicines and vaccines for all.

- Target 3.9: by 2030, substantially reduce the number of deaths and illnesses from hazardous chemicals and air, water and soil pollution and contamination.
- Target 3.a: strengthen the implementation of the World Health Organisation Framework Convention on Tobacco Control in all countries, as appropriate.
- Target 3.b: support the research and development of vaccines and medicines for the communicable and non-communicable diseases that primarily affect developing countries, provide access to affordable essential medicines and vaccines in accordance with the Doha Declaration on the TRIPS Agreement and Public Health, which affirms the right of developing countries to use to the full the provisions in the Agreement on Trade-Related Aspects of Intellectual Property Rights regarding flexibilities to protect public health and, in particular, provide access to medicines for all.
- Target 3.c: substantially increase health financing and the recruitment, development, training and retention of the health workforce in developing countries, especially in least developed countries and small island developing states.

Global Health Inequities

Despite the ambitious definition of global health and the various international commitments, global inequities persist. This is most evident when we look at life-expectancy at birth. The average life expectancy in 2024 was roughly 70 years for men and 76 years for women. However, the countries with the highest life expectancy (e.g., Monaco – 87 years, Japan – 85 years) have life expectancies that are more than 30 years higher compared to countries with the lowest life expectancy (e.g., Nigeria). Despite an average 10-year increase in life expectancy between 2000 and 2016 in the WHO African Region, the ten countries with the lowest life expectancy are exclusively located here. For example, in 2024, life expectancy in Nigeria, the most populous country on the continent, was a mere 54 years. The disparity between countries is even more cumbersome concerning healthy life expectancy at birth (meaning the years lived in good health). Other health outcome indicators, such as maternal mortality rates and child mortality rates, show a similar picture. Disparities exist not only between but also within countries where substantial gaps exist between social groups along the lines of wealth, ethnicity, literacy and migration (Beckfield et al., 2013).

The disparities between health outcomes can, to a large extent, be explained by disparities between resources for health. According to World Bank data (retrieved April 2024), the global average of spending on health per capita stood at $1,177.22, ranging from a mere $43 per capita in the poorest countries to over $5,000 in the most affluent OECD countries. In their 2019 contribution to the *Lancet*, Chang and colleagues indicate that no major changes in these trends are expected up until 2050. Also, the poorest countries in the world are more likely to rely on out of pocket expenditure for health. For households or individuals living in poverty or with limited resources, even small out-of-pocket health care expenses can represent a significant financial burden. As a consequence, they are less likely to access health care services and are more likely to face the consequences of "catastrophic health expenditure". Catastrophic health

Life expectancy, 2021

The period life expectancy[1] at birth, in a given year.

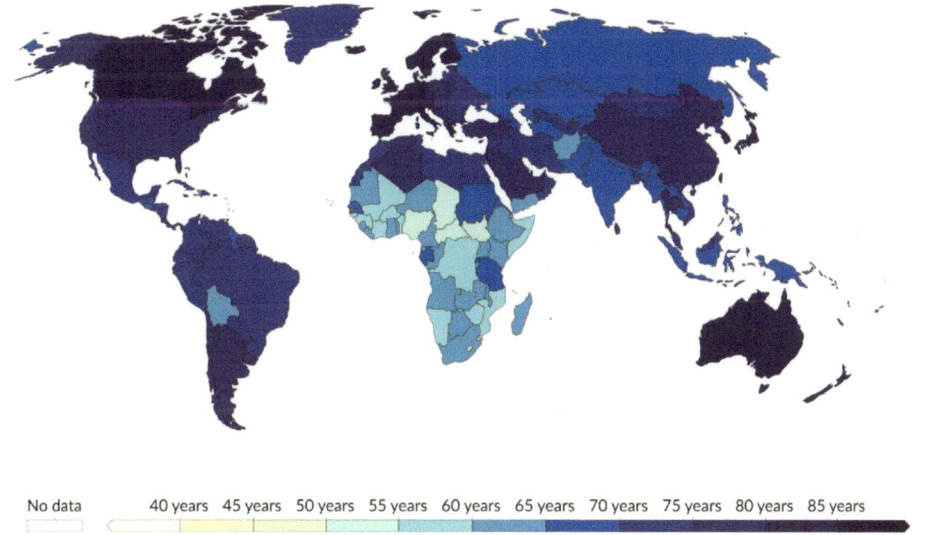

No data   40 years 45 years 50 years 55 years 60 years 65 years 70 years 75 years 80 years 85 years

Figure 2.3 Life Expectancy, 2021

Healthy life expectancy, 2019

The estimated average number of years lived free from disability or disease burden. This is based on period life expectancy[1], after adjusting for the number of years lived in less than "full health" due to disease and/or injury.

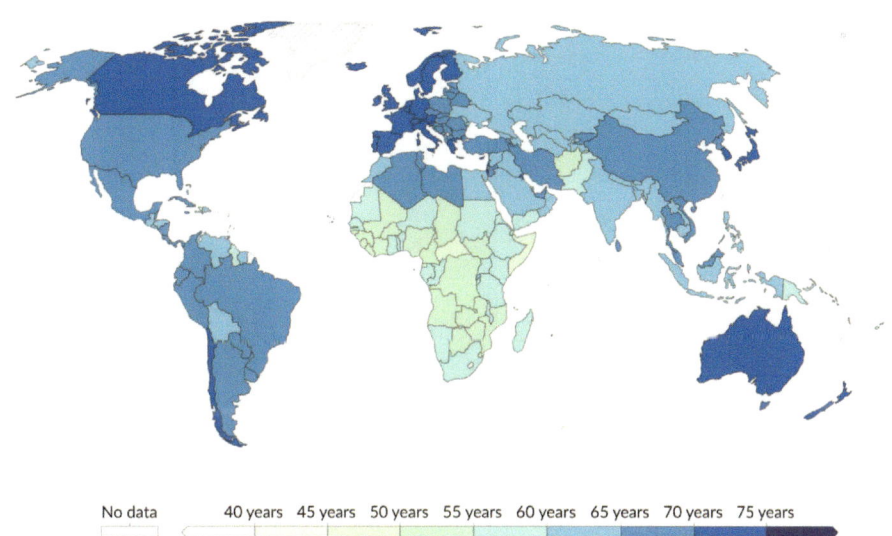

No data   40 years 45 years 50 years 55 years 60 years 65 years 70 years 75 years

Figure 2.4 Healthy Life Expectancy, 2019

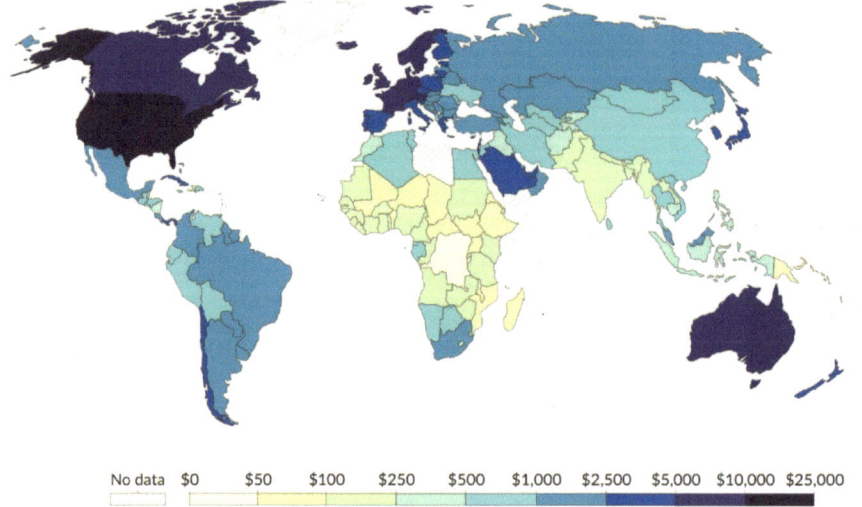

Total health expenditure per person, 2021

The sum of public and private annual health expenditure per person. This data is adjusted for differences in the cost of living between countries, but it is not adjusted for inflation.

No data $0 $50 $100 $250 $500 $1,000 $2,500 $5,000 $10,000 $25,000

Figure 2.5 Total Health Expenditure per Person, 2021

Share of out-of-pocket expenditure on health care, 2021

Out-of-pocket expenditure on healthcare as percent of total current healthcare expenditure.

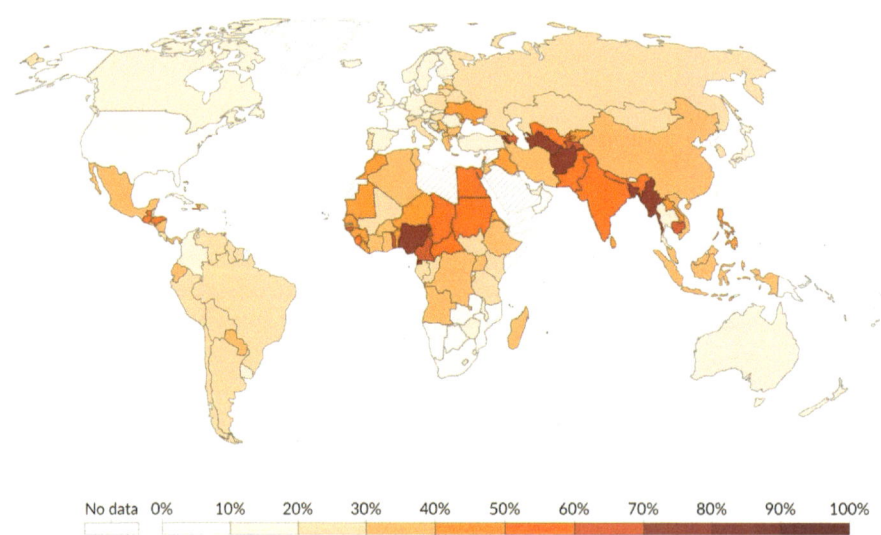

No data 0%   10%   20%   30%   40%   50%   60%   70%   80%   90%   100%

Figure 2.6 Share of Out-of-pocket Expenditure on Health care, 2021

expenditure occurs when a person or a household spends a significant portion of their income on health-related expenses, leading to financial strain, inability to access further health care and restricted their ability to afford other essential needs such as food, education and shelter. Annually, 50 million people worldwide experience catastrophic health expenditures. Therefore one of the great challenges to global health is ensuring affordable care for all. Addressing this issue necessitates the redistribution of resources for health from the rich to the poor and from the healthy to the sick.

Taking a life-course approach, it is disheartening to recognise that health inequities are perpetual. Limited access to health care, often compounded by poverty and limited access to information, impedes educational and economic opportunities in life. This, in turn, adversely impacts the health of individuals and their families, perpetuating a cycle of disadvantage. This is most profound during the so-called first 1,000 days, spanning from conception to the age of two. During this time, factors such as the mother's health status, the stress she experiences and limited access to proper nutrition can significantly impact the physical and cognitive development of the child. This heightened vulnerability increases the risk of disease and decreased intelligence later in life (e.g., Cusick & Georgieff, 2016), consequently increasing the likelihood of perpetuating a cycle of adversity across generations.

Current Challenges in Global Health

The chapter will briefly address some of the current and future challenges in global health. The examples presented are by no means exhaustive. Global health faces ongoing health challenges and is confronted with new dilemmas. While some classical global health problems have known solutions, they persist. For example, although Polio was eliminated from certain regions in the world, complete eradication remains elusive due to issues such as underfunding, political instability and increasing vaccine hesitancy. Similarly, malnutrition persists despite the global abundance of food in the world, with millions of children and pregnant women lacking access. Infectious diseases like tuberculosis continue to be a major concern, with incidence rates remaining stable and mortality stubbornly high at 1.6 million deaths annually, despite the availability of treatment regimens (WHO TB Report, 2022). This situation is further complicated by the rise of drug-resistant tuberculosis pathogens and resistant strains more broadly, exacerbating the challenge of controlling these diseases.

Prior to COVID-19, anti-microbial resistance (AMR) was the most pressing global health issue. According to the WHO, AMR continues to rank among the key global public health challenges, contributing to nearly 5 million deaths worldwide in 2019. Notably, its repercussions extend beyond health, posing a threat to the global economy through effects on international trade, health care systems and productivity. Without intervention, AMR's economic toll could soar to an estimated US$100 trillion by 2050. Its drivers are diverse and include self-medication, incorrect prescriptions, poor adherence, overuse in livestock, poor surveillance, limited production of new antibiotics due to a lack of financial incentives and restrictive access to antibiotics. Also, non-communicable-diseases (NCDs) and multimorbidity are increasing rapidly. For example, in 2017, it was estimated that globally 462 million individuals had type 2 diabetes, corresponding to 6.28% of the world's population (World Diabetes Report, 2017). This is expected to rise significantly in the coming decades. Simultaneously, there is a global rise in the prevalence of mental health disorders, cancers and cardiovascular disease. These trends are particularly worrisome for health systems in the less affluent parts of the world that are currently more geared towards dealing with acute and treatable infectious diseases.

Although global health financing has steadily increased over the past two decades, one of the largest challenges for the global health agenda is sustainable finance

(Chang et al., 2019). Financing for health is expected to grow over the coming decades, albeit at a slower pace than the past decades, with persistent disparities in per-capita health spending between countries. Also, out-of-pocket spending is projected to remain substantial in non-high-income countries; currently there are over 150 million people yearly facing catastrophic health expenditure. Many low-income countries are likely to continue relying (partly) on development assistance. In the absence of sustained new investments, improving the efficiency of health spending is essential to meet global health targets.

Although beyond the scope of this chapter, future challenges in global health will likely also relate to the effects of climate change, the "earth crisis". Planetary health addresses the broader implications of the global environmental crisis, considering how human activities are altering Earth's natural systems. This includes disturbances to biodiversity; pollution of air, water and soil; and changes in land use patterns.

Ongoing and potential armed conflict also profoundly impact global health by destroying health care infrastructure, leading to reduced access to medical care and the spread of infectious diseases (e.g., see Darrudi et al., 2022). Mental health issues rise due to violence and displacement, while chronic diseases worsen from disrupted care. Food shortages cause malnutrition, and maternal and child health deteriorate due to inadequate care. Human rights abuses also escalate, severely affecting physical and psychological health, highlighting the critical need for peace and stability. Part III of the book engages with some of the future challenges in the field of global health and human rights.

Epistemic Injustice and Decolonising Global Health

Despite its narrative of achieving equity, global health has its roots in colonial medicine and continues to face critiques that label it as "colonial" today. The notion of decolonising global health arises from enduring inequities and power imbalances between global health practitioners and researchers from the "Global North" and those from the "Global South". This is particularly evident in the prevailing donor-recipient model, where wealthy countries "give" and less affluent countries passively receive funding. This dynamic creates a significant power imbalance that dictates the agenda and implementation strategies in global health. Furthermore, local knowledge systems are often discarded; a phenomenon known as epistemicide (Bennett, 2007; de Sousa Santos, 2007; Dutta et al., 2022). This concept critiques the dominance of Western epistemologies and highlights how colonialism, globalisation and other power structures have suppressed and marginalised diverse ways of knowing. Addressing power imbalances and embedded epistemic injustices represents one of the greatest challenges within the global health system today. As outlined by Adhikari et al. (2023, p. e982) in a special issue of the *Lancet Global Health*, there is a shared vision within the decolonising global health movement:

> we envision a utopian future wherein health-care providers and researchers, regardless of country of residence or origin, receive equal opportunities in recognition; research and publishing; training; access to international travel for conferences and work; and salaries and incentives, so that every LMIC expert is considered equivalent to their high-income country (HIC) counterparts. We ultimately hope for a future in which people from every country have equal access to

quality health care, fulfilling the aspiration of universal health coverage proposed by WHO.

They point out that there should be equal opportunities within the research field, but this should also be accompanied with equal incentives and access to training. Without access to such resources, it will be very difficult to create equivalence between researchers.

Kumar and colleagues (2024) describe three intersecting dimensions of colonialism in global health that provide a perspective on how knowledge and power systems affect the practice of global health – colonialism within global health, colonisation of global health and colonialism through global health.

Colonialism within global health research refers to the significant inequities in funding for global health. Global North institutions are often favoured for grant calls explicitly or implicitly through eligibility criteria or capacity requirements. Most funding of these often short-term projects ends up being spent on salaries in the Global North, undermining long-term health systems strengthening in the Global South. For example, 82% of the Bill and Melinda Gates Foundation's grant funding to address global health challenges in 2021 went to HIC recipients. This is further exemplified and reinforced by publishing systems that favour authors from the Global North.

Colonialism of global health in turn refers to the fact that priorities for global health research (and practice) are set by institutions and even individuals from the Global North who generally favour entrepreneurship and private initiatives. Funding is more often than not directed towards technology-driven "magic bullets" (e.g., vaccines, medicines, bed nets, mobile apps), rather than systems capacity strengthening and addressing wider SDH. The investments of these "patronising" institutions are often welcomed by recipient countries; however, this often leads to reducing local investments.

Colonialism through global health refers to the question of who benefits. Kumar and colleagues (2024) argue that the asymmetric global health research and practice funding structures allow powerful states and private actors to shape research and practice in the Global South to their financial and economic advantage. These benefits stem from the commercialisation of research and publishing and market expansion imperatives, including unfair intellectual property rights and trade regimes.

To address these intersecting dimensions, it is critical to examine ideological and epistemological underpinnings of global health, to analyse the evolutionary patterns and impact of global health research and practice and to reform global health governance to deal with power imbalances. Also, achieving true power transfer and equitable partnerships in global health requires dedicating a tremendous effort to building research infrastructures.

The decolonising movement should ultimately contribute to equal partnerships and, critically, to epistemic justice. Epistemic injustice is understood as an injustice perpetuated through knowledge production – through the means of distortion, misrepresentation and mistrust – of someone's knowledge or through exclusion and forced silencing (Anderson, 2012). For example, Bhakuni and Abimbola (2021) argue that epistemic wrongs are being committed in terms of authorship practice, sensemaking practice, editorial practice and research partnership. Empirical research clearly supports this. For example, Hedt-Gauthier and colleagues (2019) analysed 7,100 published articles on health research in Africa. They found that more than 50% of all coauthors and first authors were from the country of the paper's focus. But when any coauthors were from the US, Canada and Europe, the overall representation of African authors dropped significantly, especially in the numbers of the first and last authors, in other words, keeping the African authors "stuck in the middle". Also, almost all high-ranking journals are based in the Global North.

Fricker, who coined the term epistemic injustice, argues that epistemic injustice is perpetuated in two forms, which are testimonial injustice and hermeneutical injustice. According to her, testimonial injustice is a form of prejudice through which one's knowledge is perceived as untrustworthy, epistemically lesser and misjudged. In the case of hermeneutical injustice, through marginalisation and unequal hermeneutical opportunity, people often cannot express and interpret the experience they are having in their lives (Fricker, 2017).

Naidu (2021, p. e1332) remarks that the field of global health exists because of epistemic oppression, which in turn leads to the production of intrinsically flawed knowledge:

> health issues in LMICs might be the reason for which global health exists as a field. As self-sanctioned champions of so-called tropical medicine, global health, and social medicine, scholars in HICs have shaped health in LMICs through subjective lenses, while claiming to be objective.

To address this epistemic oppression, Naidu advocates for epistemic disobedience, which involves presenting and enacting diverse perspectives, including those of "the marginalised knowers".

As a knowledge production field, global health has its epistemological roots in the fields of tropical medicine and international health which are not only the product of colonialism, but in the age of imperialism they destruct traditional knowledge and capture the knowledge production system in the Global South (Abimbola, 2018). Thereby, these knowledge systems often neglect the lived experience of communities whose issues should be at the starting point of global health practices. Thereby they perpetuate the very power imbalances they aim to address. Keshri and Bhaumik (2022) argued that academics and practitioners based in institutions situated in HICs often act as the feudal lords or "Zamindars" of global health. This metaphor describes how these individuals and institutions exert control over global health priorities, policies and resource allocation through hierarchical, feudal structures. This "feudalism" is often justified through narratives suggesting that LMICs lack the "technical skills" or "subject matter expertise" needed (Keshri & Bhaumik, 2022). This occurs through colonial and extractive attitudes, as well as policies and practices that centralise resources, expertise, data and branding within HIC-based institutions and a select few from the Global South who have access to these systems.

Therefore, the effort to decolonise global health should be accompanied by the effort to achieve epistemic justice in the field of global health. Decolonisation of global health is crucial to move towards the universal right to health and to move the universal health coverage agenda forward.

Concluding Remarks

The history and evolution of global health has been heavily influenced by colonial practices. Despite its strong connection to human rights, the field continues to be (partly) shaped by these same colonial influences today. Removing the power and knowledge inequities, as well as addressing the SDH, are critical to address the objective of global health, "improving health and achieving equity in health for all people worldwide".

Questions for Discussion

- Discuss the trends on life expectancy among the US, Kenya, India and Japan from a historical perspective. Use "Our World in Data" and/or "Gapminder" to see data visualised.
- Discuss what you find the most pressing global health challenges in your context.
- Discuss what social determinants cause the most pressing inequities in health today.
- Discuss what a human rights perspective on decolonising global health would imply.
- Discuss who should lead the decolonisation movement and what are the priority actions to undertake.
- Discuss in your institutional setting whether there are cases of epistemic injustice.

References

Abimbola, S. (2018). On the meaning of global health and the role of global health journals. *International Health*, *10*(2), 63–65.

Adhikari, S., Torres, I., & Oele, E. (2023). The way forward in decolonising global health. *The Lancet Global Health*, *11*(7), e982.

Affun-Adegbulu, C., Cosaert, T., Meudec, M., Michielsen, J., Van de Pas, R., Van Belle, S., Van De Put, W., Soors, W., Robertson, F., & Ddungu, C. (2023). Decolonisation initiatives at the institute of tropical medicine, Antwerp, Belgium: Ready for change? *BMJ Global Health*, *8*(5).

Amster, E. (2016). The Syphilitic Arab. *French Mediterraneans: Transnational and Imperial Histories*, 320–346.

Anderson, E. (2012). Epistemic justice as a virtue of social institutions. *Social Epistemology*, *26*(2), 163–173.

Beckfield, J., Olafsdottir, S., & Bakhtiari, E. (2013). Health inequalities in global context. *American Behavioral Scientist*, *57*(8), 1014–1039.

Bennett, K. (2007). Epistemicide! The tale of a predatory discourse. *The Translator*, *13*(2), 151–169.

Bhakuni, H., & Abimbola, S. (2021). Epistemic injustice in academic global health. *The Lancet Global Health*, *9*(10), e1465–e1470.

Brown, T. M., Cueto, M., & Fee, E. (2006). The World Health Organization and the transition from "international" to "global" public health. *American Journal of Public Health*, *96*(1), 62–72.

Chang, A. Y., Cowling, K., Micah, A. E., Chapin, A., Chen, C. S., Ikilezi, G., Sadat, N., Tsakalos, G., Wu, J., Younker, T., Zhao, Y., Zlavog, B. S., Abbafati, C., Ahmed, A. E., Alam, K., Alipour, V., Aljunid, S. M., Almalki, M. J., Alvis-Guzman, N., . . . Dieleman, J. L. (2019). Past, present, and future of global health financing: A review of development assistance, government, out-of-pocket, and other private spending on health for 195 countries, 1995–2050. *The Lancet*, *393*(10187), 2233–2260.

Cusick, S. E., & Georgieff, M. K. (2016). The role of nutrition in brain development: The golden opportunity of the "first 1000 days". *The Journal of Pediatrics*, *175*, 16–21.

Darrudi, A., Khoonsari, M. H. K., & Tajvar, M. (2022). Challenges to achieving universal health coverage throughout the world: A systematic review. *Journal of Preventive Medicine and Public Health*, *55*(2), 125.

de Sousa Santos, B. (2007). Beyond abyssal thinking: From global lines to ecologies of knowledges. *Review (Fernand Braudel Center)*, 45–89.

Dutta, U., Azad, A. K., Mullah, M., Hussain, K. S., & Parveez, W. (2022). From rhetorical "inclusion" toward decolonial futures: Building communities of resistance against structural violence. *American Journal of Community Psychology*, *69*(3–4), 355–368.

Fricker, M. (2017). Evolving concepts of epistemic injustice. In *The Routledge handbook of epistemic injustice* (pp. 53–60). Routledge.

Gaynes, R. P. (2023). *Germ theory: Medical pioneers in infectious diseases*. John Wiley & Sons.

Greenwood, A. (2022). Diagnosing the medical history of British imperialism. *The Lancet*, *400*(10354), 726–727.

Hedt-Gauthier, B. L., Jeufack, H. M., Neufeld, N. H., Alem, A., Sauer, S., Odhiambo, J., Boum, Y., Shuchman, M., & Volmink, J. (2019). Stuck in the middle: A systematic review of authorship in collaborative health research in Africa, 2014–2016. *BMJ Global Health*, *4*(5), e001853.

Kapilashrami, A., & Hankivsky, O. (2018). Intersectionality and why it matters to global health. *The Lancet*, *391*(10140), 2589–2591.

Keshri, V. R., & Bhaumik, S. (2022). The feudal structure of global health and its implications for decolonisation. *BMJ Global Health*, *7*(9), e010603.

Koplan, J. P., Bond, T. C., Merson, M. H., Reddy, K. S., Rodriguez, M. H., Sewankambo, N. K., & Wasserheit, J. N. (2009). Towards a common definition of global health. *The Lancet*, *373*(9679), 1993–1995.

Kumar, R., Khosla, R., & McCoy, D. (2024). Decolonising global health research: Shifting power for transformative change. *PLOS Global Public Health*, *4*(4), e0003141.

Livi-Bacci, M. (2006). The depopulation of Hispanic America after the conquest. *Population and Development Review*, *32*(2), 199–232.

Naidu, T. (2021). Says who? Northern ventriloquism, or epistemic disobedience in global health scholarship. *The Lancet Global Health*, *9*(9), e1332–e1335.

Salm, M., Ali, M., Minihane, M., & Conrad, P. (2021). Defining global health: Findings from a systematic review and thematic analysis of the literature. *BMJ Global Health*, *6*(6), e005292.

Tulchinsky, T. H. (2018). Bismarck and the long road to universal health coverage. *Case Studies in Public Health*, *131*.

Vinten-Johansen, P., Brody, H., Paneth, N., Rachman, S., Rip, M., & Zuck, D. (2003). *Cholera, chloroform, and the science of medicine: A life of John Snow*. Oxford University Press.

Vogt, M. (2022). Development postcolonial: A critical approach to understanding SDGs in the perspective of Christian social ethics. *Global Sustainability*, *5*, e4.

For Further Reading

Meier, B. M., & Gostin, L. O. (Eds.). (2018). *Human rights in global health: Rights-based governance for a globalizing world*. Oxford University Press.

Merson, M. H., Black, R. E., & Mills, A. J. (2011). *Global health: Diseases, programs, systems, and policies*. Jones & Bartlett Learning.

Ndlovu-Garshenia, S. J. (2018). *Epistemic freedom in Africa: Deprovincialization and decolonisation*. Routledge.

Sethia, B., & Kumar, P. (Eds.). (2018). *Essentials of global health*. Elsevier Health Sciences.

CHAPTER 3

The Right to Health

Cees J. Hamelink

Introduction

Health and human rights are related in three ways.

1. Within health care systems, policies and practices may affect the safeguarding of human rights such as the right to health, the right to autonomy and privacy and the right to freedom of information.
2. The respect of human rights such as the right to education, to safe drinking water and to adequate housing may directly affect people's health.
3. Human rights violations such as arbitrary detention or torture have a direct effect on people's health.

In this chapter we shall look at the development of the health–human rights relation; study the right to health and social conditionalities of health; and address the institutionalisation of health care, moral choice, the role of the UN Special Rapporteurs on the Right to Health and the need for human rights education.

Learning Objectives

After studying this chapter you will be able to:

■ Explain the development of the international right to health and the role of the UN system with regard to this right
■ Discuss the significance and scope of the right to health
■ Identify essential social conditionalities related to the right to health
■ Discuss the right to health in relation to the autonomy of the patient
■ Understand the need of human rights education for health workers

A Definition of Health and UN Human Rights Provisions

In a far-sighted way, the WHO defined health in its 1946 constitution as "A state of complete physical, mental and social well-being". The UN community has provided for

DOI: 10.4324/9781003408765-5

the realisation of this definition a basic set of international human rights provisions in the following instruments.

Universal Declaration of Human Rights

In 1948 the UDHR proposed (in Article 25) that everyone should have the right to a standard of living adequate for the health and well-being of himself and of his family, including food, clothing, housing and medical care. Added to this, the declaration provided that "Motherhood and childhood are entitled to special care and assistance".

Although the declaration is not a legally binding instrument, over the years it has gained the force of customary law which means that its entitlements became universally accepted as essential moral principles.

International Covenant on Economic, Social and Cultural Rights

In 1966, the International Covenant on Economic, Social and Cultural Rights (ICESCR) codified the health provision of the UDHR into binding law for the UN member states that ratified the covenant (presently 171 member states have done so). Article 12 of the ICESCR provides for "The right to the enjoyment of the highest attainable standard of physical and mental health".

Alma Ata

In 1978, the World Health Organisation Alma Ata "health for all" conference focussed particularly on health care in low- and middle-income countries. In its final declaration, the conference identified primary health care as the key to the attainment of the goal of Health for All. The conference reaffirmed that health is a fundamental human right and that the attainment of the highest possible level of health is a most important world-wide social goal whose realisation requires the action of many other social and economic sectors in addition to the health sector. The conference also declared that people have a right and duty to participate individually and collectively in the planning and implementation of their health care. The Alma Ata declaration also stated that

> an acceptable level of health for all the people of the world by the year 2000 can be attained through a fuller and better use of the world's resources, a considerable part of which is now spent on armaments and military conflicts. A genuine policy of independence, peace, détente, and disarmament could and should release additional resources that could well be devoted to peaceful aims and in particular to the acceleration of social and economic development of which primary health care, as an essential part, should be allotted its proper share.

Crucial Moments

In spite of these moral and legal articulations, the domains of human rights protection and the care for public health remained for a long time separate fields. This is somewhat understandable since public health and human rights have different foci. Whereas human rights promotors tend to concentrate on the protection of individual interests, public health workers address issues of public interest. There can be serious clashes between these interests when – for example – the protection of public welfare demands restrictions on the behaviour of individuals. It was only in 1987 that Jonathan Mann (a medical doctor working for the HIV/AIDS programme of the WHO) brought human rights and human health together. He did that through his plea to protect the human rights of AIDS patients. This was a first decisive phase in the development of the health–human rights relationship. In 1993, Jonathan Mann set up with his colleagues the François-Xavier Bagnoud Centre on Health and Human Rights at the Harvard School of Public Health and launched the *Health and Human Rights Journal*. This journal has played a critical role in educating and raising awareness about health and human rights and situating health and human rights squarely within the movements that demand global recognition of health as a human right. Mann and his colleagues explained in *Health and Human Rights: A reader* that "modern human rights is a civilizational achievement, a historic effort to identify and agree upon what governments should not do to people and what they should assure to all".

A crucial second moment, also in 1993, was the World Conference on Human Rights, held in Vienna, which sent out a call for the universality, indivisibility and interdependence of all human rights and fostered a global deepening of the discourse on economic and social rights. This was followed by then UN Secretary General Kofi Annan's plea to integrate human rights across the UN system. Together, these two developments fostered a global recognition and institutionalisation of economic and social rights and the right to health in particular. Since then, desk officers on human rights have been appointed at WHO, UNFPA and other entities, and normative unpacking of these issues has been undertaken by UN Treaty Monitoring Bodies.

The third moment was the appointment of the first UN Special Rapporteur on the Right to Health in 2002, which spurred advances in the normative development of health as a human right. Similar trends can be seen outside the multilateral system with the establishment of the People's Health Movement in 2000, numerous national level litigations with claims based on the right to health and the mainstream human rights organisations, such as Amnesty International and Human Rights Watch, who expanded their mandates to include health and human rights.

The Right to Health

Health and human rights, including the right to health, was on the WHO agenda until 1953, when a change of leadership effectively suspended for many years its serious and sustained consideration within the organisation. In 1993, the WHO published Rebecca Cook's "Human Rights in Relation to Women's Health", which raised issues that contributed not only to the World Conference on Human Rights (1993) – for which it was written – but also to the International Conference on Population and Development (1994) and the Fourth World Conference on Women (1995). Four years later, the WHO held a two-day informal consultation on health and human rights which the chairperson described as "the first meeting at WHO to be convened specifically to address health and human rights". In one of the meeting's key papers, Julia Hausermann presented a conceptual framework for the right to health.

In 2002 the WHO accepted, after much deliberation, the notion of a "right to health", and the UN General Assembly appointed a special rapporteur to monitor the right to health. The mandate of the rapporteur includes to investigate the positive obligations that government policies imply for the right to health (among others the provision of information and resources that guarantee that also in privatised health care human rights are respected) and to investigate negative obligations that governments have, like not torturing people or not invading their privacies.

What, then, does this right to health entitle people to? To be healthy? To have good genes? This right makes little sense in its literal interpretations. No one can have a legal right to good health and claim the parallel state obligation to provide this. States have little influence on genetic factors. The right to health is therefore usually seen as the entitlement to an environment which enables the attainment of the highest achievable standard of health. This means that care facilities and services must exist including the provision of safe drinking water, good sanitation, trained medical staff and essential drugs. It also means that attention should be given to essential factors in an environment that facilitate the right to health such as education, income, employment, housing and protection against violence.

The AAAQ Yardstick

Health care must be **available, accessible and affordable** and on a non-discriminatory basis. These interrelated elements essential to the right to health have been highlighted in General Comment no. 14 of the OHCHR. Information about how to obtain health care services should be freely provided. Health care facilities and services should also be **acceptable** which means that they should be culturally appropriate, sensitive to gender and age and respectful of ethical requirements such as doctor–patient confidentiality. Beyond the four A's, the right to health requires that health services and facilities should operate in accordance with medical and human rights **quality**. This implies that health facilities and services should implement the guiding normative principles of the universal human rights regime. These are:

■ Respect for inherent human **dignity**. This means there should be no humiliating treatment in health care. Patients should not be seen as files, cases or numbers but as agents that participate in the process of diagnosis and treatment.

■ Recognition of **equality**. This means there should be no discrimination in access to and affordability of health services.

■ Recognition of human **autonomy**. This means that there should be no non-consensual medical intervention. Informed consent should be a crucial principle in health care. Patients should have the space to make their own choices.

■ Protection of **security**. This means that there should be no non-consensual interference with physical, mental and moral integrity. Moreover, extreme care and caution should be exercised in providing medication, and the testing and approving of new types of medication should be monitored by independent professional bodies.

Social Conditionalities of Health

The human rights approach to health was a switch from the dominant biomedical model on health. Although the biomedical model remains powerful, the human rights approach increasingly emphasised the social conditionalities of health (see also Chapter 2).

Such conditionalities include, as was mentioned earlier,

> access to safe and potable water and adequate sanitation, an adequate supply of safe food, nutrition and housing, healthy occupation and environmental conditions, and access to health-related education and information. A further important aspect is the participation of the population in all health-related decision-making at the community, national and international levels.
>
> *(OHCHR, CESCR General comment No. 14, 2000)*

The emerging rights-based approach to health is no longer based upon charity but on a legal entitlement and on the remedy of its violation. This implies the need to analyse root causes of human rights violations, listen to the "victims" and use their experiences and knowledge, see that they are agents of change and self-empowerment, establish accountability for those who violate human rights and hold the perpetrators culpable. Essential conditionalities can be identified: urbanisation, inequality and global proliferation of risks.

Urbanisation

The world has never before known so many cities and never such large cities as the massive conurbations of more than 20 million people that are now gaining ground in Asia, Latin America and Africa. Many of these cities have populations larger than entire countries. The population of Greater Mumbai (which will soon achieve megacity status), for instance, is already larger than the total population of Norway and Sweden combined.

The quality and sustainability of life in the world's cities will largely depend upon the ways in which the urbanites manage to co-exist with each other. The way cities structure and manage their public space is obviously essential to any effort to enhance social interaction among urbanites. In addition to the management of the physical environment, there are also economic and socio-cultural elements that enhance or obstruct urban social interaction. Much will depend on whether urban populations will be able to cope with such city characteristic as heterogeneity. The city is a place of heterogeneity; a place of differences and dealing with heterogeneity is exceedingly difficult for many people.

The city is also characterised by the tremendous speed of its movements and interactions. Social interactions demand time. For most city dwellers this means that they have to learn the art of slowing down. Much of urban interaction is mindless. Running without seeing faces, passing others as strangers in the night, without feelings of responsibility towards others, speeding along the urban routes in cocoons that broadcast the signal that I don't mind you, please don't mind me! It is more characteristic of urban life than of village life that numerous bystanders see a fellow human being beaten and kicked and don't intervene. They may even complain if other onlookers stand in their line of sight.

Inequality

A standard feature of today's world is inequality in the access to resources, the experience of recognition and the distribution of power.

The inequality of resources can be illustrated with the observation that the 600 million best off people have 60 times the income of the 600 million worst off or that for 1.2 billion people there is no access to safe drinking water. In today's global economy some 20% of the world's population have 80% of the global income. Worldwide inequalities in the distribution of income and capital are on the increase. There are no signs that the affluent believe that they have a responsibility for global distributive justice (Pogge, 2002).

Worldwide people's dignity is respected in highly unequal ways as the persisting discriminatory treatment of women; of the Lesbian, Gay, Bisexual, Transgender, Queer and Intersex + community (LGBTQI+); of disabled people, older people and people of colour illustrates. Forms of social division around disability and sexual orientation are a reality around the world. In the case of fractures between abled and disabled people there are practices of discrimination (like unequal treatment regarding employment) and exclusion (a.o. from social activities or public transportation). "Disabled people are disadvantaged because they belong to a group that is the object of pervasive institutionalised discrimination" (Hyde quoted by Bradley, 235).

In authoritarian countries but also in democracies power of decision-making is very unequally distributed. This is also – around the globe – the case at work and in the family. Global health issues occur in a deeply hierarchical and unequal set of power relations and are embedded in structural relationships that rob many people of their fundamental human rights and that manage to create a culture of denial and silence about these abuses.

Global Proliferation of Risks

Ulrich Beck (1992) has coined the notion of the "risk society". An important dimension of the context of global health is that we live in a global risk society. Human security is threatened by warfare (nuclear, biological and chemical), terrorism, organised crime, changes in the environment (increasing ultraviolet radiation, rising temperatures, disappearance of rain forests, shortage of drinking water, desertification, depletion of fossil fuels, decreasing biodiversity), carcinogen ingredients in food supplies, pollution by poisonous materials (acid rain, chemical products from insecticides or deodorants), series of natural disasters (asteroids, comets, volcanoes or tornados) and genetic experiments. There is hate speech around the world that incites people to ethnic, racial and religious violence. There is the advertising discourse (Ad-Speech) that persuades people to indulge in a consumption fever that puts a dangerous burden on the planet's sustainability. There are news reports in the mass media that do little to help people understand the world they live in as they frame issues in ways that serve the interests of small, political and economic elites. Also, there are developments in information/communication technology (ICT) that facilitate an unprecedented invasion in people's private lives and that create very vulnerable societies. Added to this there are the combined innovations in robotics, artificial intelligence, nanotechnology and biomedical technology that fly humanity – blindly – towards a future that may not need human beings anymore.

Social Structures of Health Injustice

The Brazilian pedagogue and philosopher Paolo Freire introduced the concept of "conscientization" or consciousness-raising to explain how social structures cause injustice (Freire, 1972). Conscious-raising involves discovering that evil not only is present in the hearts of powerful individuals who muck things up for the rest of us but is embedded in the very structures of society, so that these structures, and not just individuals who work within them, must be changed if the world is to change.

(Brown, 1993, p. 45)

These structures are often referred to as key elements of the "neo-liberal capitalism" that emerged in the early 1980s with the large scale privatisation and liberalisation of such social services as telecommunications (Chapman, 2016).

There is a very obvious, persistent and explosive worldwide fracture between the rich who continue to profit from economic growth and the poor who are facing economic stagnation (World Inequality Report, 2018). This global fracture has different sets of rules for the winners and losers. Governments bail big banks out, whereas ordinary citizens lose their houses when they cannot foot their bills. Globally, austerity policies have mainly aggravated social polarisation. These policies have made "women, ethnic minorities, the young, the old, the disabled . . . the losers and the international super-rich and national elite classes have been the winners, and the beneficiaries of other people's suffering" (Bradley, 2016, p. 268). Various calculations by different authors seem to usually end with the conclusion that a small percentage of the world population (3–5%) has control over 50% of the world's wealth. A small group of the very rich claim an ever larger part of global income and capital. According to the Global Wealth Report 2021, published by Credit Suisse, there was a substantial worldwide increase in wealth inequality during 2020. The wealth distribution pyramid in 2020 shows that the richest group of the adult population (1.1%) owned 45.8% of the total wealth. When compared to the 2013 wealth distribution pyramid, an overall increase of 4.8% can be seen in wealth inequality. This growing gap is framed by many conservative politicians and corporate media as normal (Wysong & Perrucci, 2017). In this frame, doing more with less is the "new normal". People should accept austerity budgets and widening inequalities "between wealthy and Average Americans, with regard to wealth, income, health care, employment and educational opportunities". Wysong and Perruci argue that the new normal of deep equality should not be accepted. Against the corporate media "new normal" narrative that obscures real differences, inequalities and fractures stands the "structural reality" narrative.

For us, the term structural realities narrative refers to a general story line that views origins, causes, dimensions, and consequences of current economic, political, and social inequalities as growing out of actions and policies shaped and implemented by powerful social structures such as large corporations and federal government.

(ibidem, 12)

These structures create the conditions that make the universal realisation of a state of complete physical, mental and social well-being impossible.

Health care problems cannot be resolved by health policies and practices alone but need socio-political thinking and acting that is inspired by notions of distributive justice. Genuine healing demands societal healing. It can be argued that the international human rights regime with all its shortcomings provides a basis for a universal enjoyment of the right to health. The emerging rights-based approach to health is no longer based upon charity but on a legal entitlement and on the remedy of its violation. Resulting from this there should be a solid analysis of root causes of social injustice. Poverty should be seen as a human rights violation. It is essential to listen to the victims of human rights violations so that their experiences and knowledge can be used. It should be understood that those victims are agents of change. Space should be created for their self-empowerment. Lastly, it is critical that there is accountability for those who violate human rights and that the perpetrators are held culpable.

In short: health should be located within a larger political project that seeks to develop a society that is governed not only by the rule of law but by the humanistic ideal of fundamental fairness. In Chapter 13 of this book we provide a method than can contribute to such societal change processes.

The Autonomous Patient

The right to health includes the freedom of people to make choices about their own health. This means that states, although they have the obligation to maximise the conditions under which people can enjoy health, cannot impose restrictions on the autonomy of people even for their own good (Tobin, 2012). This results in an ongoing tension between individual autonomy and collective interest. To deal with this, the legitimate restriction of individual rights for the good of public health have been worked out in international human rights law. In cases where restrictive measures address the protection of public health, the major considerations are necessity, proportionality and reasonability.

The Role of the European Convention on Human Rights and Fundamental Freedoms

In the European Convention on Human Rights and Fundamental Freedoms (ECHR) Article 5 has strengthened the legal position of psychiatric patients. It rendered involuntary institutionalisation only admissible in case of "true mental disorder of a degree warranting compulsory confinement" (ECHR, October 1979). And additionally, "special procedural safeguards may prove called for in order to protect the interests of persons who, on account of their mental disabilities are not fully capable of acting for themselves" (Ibidem). By 1992 the European Court on Human Rights had provided that cases of compulsory admission call for "increased vigilance in reviewing whether the Convention has been complied with" and "the Court must satisfy itself that the medical necessity has been convincingly shown to exist" (European Court, September 1992).

The increasing use of mobile health technologies, particularly of so-called health apps, can contribute to patient autonomy by giving more control over the process of diagnosis and treatment. There are also risks for the protection of personal privacy. The separate data about health indicators such as nutrition, weight or use of alcohol create a complete profile of people's health and health risks. In this context, Article 8 of the European Convention which provides for the right to privacy is crucial. The European Court has emphasised that, following this Article, the use of modern technology should be weighed against the interests of the individual.

The international human rights regime provides that the medical profession must respect the choices of the autonomous patient. It is, however, necessary to make a mindful footnote here. The autonomous patient may also be the lonesome patient: left alone to make existential choices. It could be that the patient would prefer to decide together with a circle of trusted and loved persons. Or it could be that the medical professional should reach out to patients and be with them – in a non-paternalistic but caring way – when crucial choices have to be made. It is also essential that autonomous choices are made on the basis of relevant and comprehensible information.

The Commercialisation of Health Care

Around the world health care services are – as part of neo-liberal economic policies – provided by private commercial parties. This raises the issue of the human rights obligations of private health care providers and the question of whether this leads to better health care and what it means for the accessibility and affordability of health services to poor segments of the population. Will privatisation increase or decrease societal inequalities in access to health care? Since international human rights law does not address the specific of national economic systems, the privatisation and commercialisation of health services is not prohibited. However, national states should require such services to meet the obligation to contribute to the progressive realisation of the right to health. This implies that "states are not exempt from their obligations under human rights law when they outsource or privatise services that impact the realisation of the right to health" (Tobin & Barrett, 2020, p. 80).

Universal Health Coverage (UHC)

Since the 1978 Declaration of Alma Ata on primary care (WHO, n.d.), a core issue in the global policies of the World Health Organisation has become Universal Health Coverage. The Declaration proclaims that governments have a responsibility for the health of their people which can be fulfilled only by the provision of adequate health and social measures. It states that a main social target of governments, international organisations, and the whole world community in the coming decades should be the attainment by all peoples of the world by the year 2000 a level of health that will permit them to lead a socially and economically productive life. Primary health care is the key to attaining this target as part of development in the spirit of social justice. Even by the year 2024 this target – now also included in the UN Sustainable Development Goals (UN, n.d.) – has not been reached.

In the 2019 UN Declaration "Universal Health Coverage: Moving Together to Build a Healthier World" the right to health can be seen as the normative cornerstone of the global consensus on UHC. An important feature of UHC is obviously to provide health care to all without financial hindrances. Around the world countries deal with this challenge in different ways. There are universal public health care systems (like in the UK, Canada and Australia), private insurance systems (like in the USA) and a mixed system of public and private insurance. As health insurance differs around the world, the key question remains what mode of funding with ever more expensive health care can guarantee a rights-based universal health coverage. However, redistribution of resources between the rich and the poor – and between the sick and the healthy – is essential to ensure financial risk protection.

The UN Rapporteurs on the Right to Health

Key Developments in the United Nations

In addition to a growing scholarly literature since 1999–2000, there have been significant health and human rights developments in the UN. The post-1999–2000 UN developments may be divided into two groups: those that focus on the right to health and those with wider formulations, such as human rights-based approaches to health, which include the right to health. Much can be learnt from the reports of the UN Special Rapporteurs. In 2007, the Human Rights Council asked the Special Rapporteur to prepare a report on health systems and the right to health. At that time, there was scarce guidance from the treaty bodies or elsewhere on this topic, and so the rapporteur turned to basic principles, analogous practice and extensive consultations and began to fill this jurisprudential gap. The mandate of the Special Rapporteur on the right of everyone to the enjoyment of the highest attainable standard of physical and mental health was originally established by the Commission on Human Rights in April 2002 by resolution 2002/31. Subsequent to the replacement of the Commission by the Human Rights Council in June 2006, the mandate was endorsed and extended by a series of Human Rights Council resolutions.

The scope of the mandate of the Special Rapporteur on the right of everyone to the enjoyment of the highest attainable standard of physical and mental health was established by resolution 6/29 of 14 December 2007 and consists of the following elements:

> to gather, request, receive and exchange information from all relevant sources, including Governments, intergovernmental and non-governmental organizations, on the realisation of the right of everyone to the enjoyment of the highest attainable standard of physical and mental health, as well as policies designed to achieve the health-related Millennium Development Goals;
>
> To develop a regular dialogue and discuss possible areas of cooperation with all relevant actors, including Governments, relevant United Nations bodies, specialized agencies and programmes, in particular the World Health Organization and the Joint United Nations Programme on HIV/AIDS, as well as non-governmental organizations and international financial institutions;
>
> To report on the status, throughout the world, of the realisation of the right of everyone to the enjoyment of the highest attainable standard of physical and mental health and on developments relating to this right, including on laws, policies and good practices most beneficial to its enjoyment and obstacles encountered domestically and internationally to its implementation;
>
> to make recommendations on appropriate measures to promote and protect the realisation of the right of everyone to the enjoyment of the highest attainable standard of physical and mental health, with a view to supporting States' efforts to enhance public health; To submit an annual report to the Human Rights Council and an interim report to the General Assembly on its activities, findings, conclusions and recommendations.

The Human Rights Council further encourages the Special Rapporteur:

> to continue to explore how efforts to realize the right of everyone to the enjoyment of the highest attainable standard of physical and mental health can reinforce poverty reduction strategies;

To continue the analysis of the human rights dimensions of the issues of neglected diseases and diseases particularly affecting developing countries, and also the national and international dimensions of those issues;

To continue to pay particular attention to the identification of good practices for the effective operationalization of the right of everyone to the enjoyment of the highest attainable standard of physical and mental health;

To continue to apply a gender perspective in her/his work and to pay special attention to the needs of children and other vulnerable and marginalised groups in the realisation of the right of everyone to the enjoyment of the highest attainable standard of physical and mental health;

To pay due attention to the rights of persons with disabilities in the context of the realisation of the right of everyone to the enjoyment of the highest attainable standard of physical and mental health;

To continue to pay attention to sexual and reproductive health as an integral element of the right of everyone to the enjoyment of the highest attainable standard of physical and mental health;

To continue to avoid in her/his work any duplication or overlapping with the work, competence and mandate of other international bodies active in health issues;

To submit proposals that could help the realisation of the health-related Millennium Development Goals.

Since 2002, UN Special Rapporteurs on the right to health have applied the treaties and general comments to many themes, states and other duty bearers. When rapporteurs have encountered specific issues on which the existing jurisprudence gives no or scant guidance, they have offered their interpretations of the international right to health. UN agencies have adopted increasingly detailed guidance on how to operationalise human rights, for example, in relation to HIV/AIDS, tuberculosis, maternal mortality, under-five mortality, contraceptive information and services and clinical management of female genital mutilation. This has required agencies to interpret and apply treaties, general comments and other jurisprudence, sometimes weighing the available evidence as part of their interpretative process. None of these initiatives is above criticism but, at least, as John Harrington and Maria Stuttaford put it, a "beginning has been made" to provide treaty provisions with detailed normative and operational content (Harrington & Stuttaford, 2010). In recent years the Special Rapporteurs reported on the right to mental health, deprivation of liberty and the right to health, corruption and the right to health, sports and healthy lifestyles as contributing factors to the right to health and the right to health in early childhood as a right to survival and development. All the reports can be found online!

Human Rights Education for Health Care Professionals
Health care workers can contribute to the protection of human rights standards by:

Providing care without discrimination
Respecting the autonomy and dignity of patients
Respecting patient confidentiality
Obtaining informed consent before treatment.

Health workers may experience pressures from inside or outside their direct work environment that form obstacles to the protection of human rights such as:

Institutional rules and regulations
Unequal power relations
Personal beliefs and convictions
Health laws and policies
Lack of necessary resources.

The UN Special Rapporteur has also begun to promote the uptake of health care worker education based on human rights principles. From the selection of students to the curricula taught, the location of training and subsequent employment within health systems, he promotes the impact that human rights-based approaches to medical education can have on the health care workforce. Integration of human rights into health education can help health care workers overcome their own inherent discriminatory behaviours and attitudes. The Special Rapporteur does not intend to replicate the global effort to – and volume of literature on – the health care workforce crisis but to show the impact that human rights-based approaches to medical and other health education can make. He identifies features of current health education that limit the capacity of the health care workforce to function effectively and to play its crucial role in promoting, respecting and fulfilling the right to physical and mental health. He presents some structural elements that shape the capacity of the health care workforce to fulfil states' right-to-health obligations to make health care available, accessible, acceptable and of good quality, while also applying a right-to-health framework to health care workers themselves in order to identify issues that can enhance or restrict their ability to perform well.

Human rights education (HRE) is a recently established field of educational theory and practice gaining increased attention and significance across the globe. This effort, which has gained momentum since the early 1990s, has spawned a growing body of educational theory, practice and research that often intersects with activities in other fields of educational study, such as citizenship education, peace education, anti-racism education, holocaust/genocide education, education for sustainable development and education for intercultural understanding. Inter-governmental organisations, including the UN and regional human rights entities such as the Council of Europe, have promoted human rights education in policies and practices. There is now a permanent and ongoing World Program for HRE (UN, 2005), and in 2011 the UN General Assembly passed the Declaration on Human Rights Education and Training. From the UN point of view, knowledge about human rights by all actors in society is fundamental to the virtuous cycle of people knowing and claiming their rights and governments being held accountable for their human rights promises.

From the UN Declaration on Human Rights Education and Training (2011)
1. Human rights education and training comprises all educational, training, information, awareness-raising and learning activities aimed at promoting universal respect for and observance of all human rights and fundamental freedoms and thus

contributing, inter alia, to the prevention of human rights violations and abuses by providing persons with knowledge, skills and understanding and developing their attitudes and behaviours, to empower them to contribute to the building and promotion of a universal culture of human rights.

2. Human rights education and training encompasses: (a) Education about human rights, which includes providing knowledge and understanding of human rights norms and principles, the values that underpin them and the mechanisms for their protection; (b) Education through human rights, which includes learning and teaching in a way that respects the rights of both educators and learners; (c) Education for human rights, which includes empowering persons to enjoy and exercise their rights and to respect and uphold the rights of others.

HRE should ultimately result in learners being motivated to promote and protect human rights, and knowing that human rights and human rights principles will be experienced as relevant to their daily lives. The latter HRE aim alludes to a behavioural change approach (from Tibbitts, 2002).

Human Rights-based Health Care

Human rights-based health care also raises the issue of human responsibilities in relation to health care. When Mahatma Gandhi was asked what he thought of a declaration of human rights, he answered in a letter to the director general of UNESCO (25 May of 1947) "I learned from my illiterate but wise mother that rights stem from duties well done". In 1997, the Interaction Council proposed the Universal Declaration of Human Responsibilities (appended). The notion of human responsibility can be seen as a central theme in human rights education. Human rights, however valuable, are state-centric and state dependent. This means that the right holder is a passive agent and dependent upon state authorities primarily for the protection of their rights. The rights concept is also problematic when it comes to rights of animals, rivers or mountains. Those rights automatically translate into human responsibilities since the subjects of these rights cannot claim their realisation. Human responsibility is a more active notion since those who have responsibilities have moral agency to exercise these responsibilities. Human rights imply the dependency of rights bearers upon state-centred institutions. Human responsibilities imply the active agency of the responsibility-bearers.

An interesting exercise would be to take Article 25 of the Universal Declaration of Human Rights (UN, 1948) and formulate the text as an article in the Universal Declaration of Human Responsibilities (see Appendix A).

> Everyone has the right to a standard of living adequate for the health and well-being of himself and of his family, including food, clothing, housing and medical care and necessary social services, and the right to security in the event of unemployment, sickness, disability, widowhood, old age or other lack of livelihood in circumstances beyond his control.
>
> *(UDHR, Article 25)*

Concluding Remarks

The right to health provides not the right to be healthy but the entitlement to the institutions, structures and resources that contribute to an optimal state of health. No one can have a legal right to good health and claim the parallel state obligation to provide this. States have little influence on genetic factors. The right to health is therefore seen as the entitlement to an environment which enables the attainment of the highest achievable standard of health. This means that care facilities and services must exist including the provision of safe drinking water, good sanitation, trained medical staff and essential drugs. Health care must be affordable and accessible on a non-discriminatory basis. Information about how to obtain health care services should be freely provided. Health care facilities and services should be acceptable, which means that they should be culturally appropriate, sensitive to gender and age and respectful of ethical requirements such as doctor–patient confidentiality. Beyond the four A requirements (availability, accessibility, affordability and acceptability), health services and facilities should operate in accordance with the quality principles of professional health care and human rights standards. Health facilities and services should implement the guiding normative principles of the international human rights regime. These are:

- Respect for inherent human dignity. This means there should be no humiliating treatment.
- Recognition of equality. This means there should be no discrimination.
- Recognition of human autonomy. This means there should be no non-consensual interference with independent choice.
- Protection of security. This means there should be no non-consensual interference with physical, mental and moral integrity.

Questions for Discussion
- Discuss the core obligations for countries in terms of the protection of the right to health.
- Discuss whether there are individual obligations towards the protection of the right to health.
- Discuss which violations of human rights have serious impact on public health.
- Discuss what would be the key features of a convivial health care institution.
- Discuss whether the current global economic order poses a serious threat to the right to health.
- Discuss how the principles of a rights-based approach to health care could be part of a national health policy. Those principles are
  - Participation of the population in the provision of health services
  - Improvement of health services in a non-discriminatory way
  - Promotion of transparency
  - Accountability of public actors for their action on health care
  - Adequate funding for capacity development
  - Accountability of non-state actors
- "Human rights education for health care professionals improves health care". Discuss how and why more knowledge about human rights would or would not contribute to better practices in health care.

Note

1 *Health and Human Rights* is an online, open-access publication, supported by the FXB Harvard School of Public Health and partners at the Dornsife School of Public Health, Drexel University, as well as the Harvard Health and Human Rights Consortium.

References

Beck, U. (1992). *Risk society.* Sage.

Bradley, H. (2016). *Fractured identities: Changing patterns of inequality.* Polity Press.

Brown, R. M. (1993). *Liberation theology.* John Knox Press.

Chapman, A. (2016). *Global health, human rights and the challenge of neoliberal policies.* Cambridge University Press.

Freire, P. (1972). *Pedagogy of the oppressed.* Penguin Editions.

Harrington, J., & Stuttaford, M. (2010). Introduction. In J. Harrington & M. Stuttaford (Eds.), *Global health and human rights: Legal and philosophical perspectives.* Routledge.

Pogge, T. (2002). *World poverty and human rights.* Polity Press.

Tibbitts, F. (2002). Emerging models for human rights education. *International Review of Education, 48*(3–4), 159–171.

Tobin, J. (2012). *The right to health in international law.* Oxford University Press.

Tobin, J., & Barrett, D. (2020). The right to health and health-related human rights. In L. O. Gostin & B. M. Meier (Eds.), *Foundations of global health & human rights* (pp. 67–87). Oxford University Press.

UN. (1948). *Universal Declaration of Human Rights.* https://www.un.org/en/about-us/universal-declaration-of-human-rights

UN. (2000). *E/C.12/2000/4: General Comment No. 14 on the highest attainable standard of health (2000).* The Committee on Economic, Social and Cultural Rights.

UN. (2005). *World Programme for Human Rights Education.* https://www.ohchr.org/en/resources/educators/human-rights-education-training/world-programme-human-rights-education

UN. (n.d.). *The 17 goals.* https://sdgs.un.org/goals

WHO. (n.d.). *Social determinants of health: WHO called to return to the declaration of Alma-Ata.* https://www.who.int/teams/social-determinants-of-health/declaration-of-alma-ata

Wysong, E., & Perrucci, R. (2017). *Deep inequality: Understanding the new normal and how to challenge it.* Rowman and Littlefield.

For Further Reading

Health and Human Rights Journal.[1] This journal began publication in 1994 under the editorship of Jonathan Mann. Paul Farmer, co-founder of Partners In Health, assumed the editorship in 2007. *Health and Human Rights* provides an inclusive forum for action-oriented dialogue among human rights practitioners.

Farmer, P. (2005). *Pathologies of power: Health, human rights and the new war on the poor.* University of California Press.

Gruskin, S., Mills, E., & Tarantola, D. (2015). History, principles, and practice of health and human rights. *The Lancet, 370*(2007).

Hunt, P. (2016). Interpreting the international right to health in a human rights-based approach to health. *Health and Human Rights Journal, 18*(2), 109–130.

Illich, I. (1974). *Medical nemesis.* Calder & Boyars.

The International Federation of Health and Human Rights Organisations. (2012). *Steps for change: A human rights action guide for health workers.* https://www.ifhhro.org/wp-content/uploads/2017/09/ifhhro_steps_for_change_en.pdf

Toebes, B. (1999). *The right to health as a human right in international law.* Intersentia.

Venkatapuram, S. (2011). *Health justice: An argument from the capabilities approach.* Polity Press.

Appendix A

A Universal Declaration of Human Responsibilities. Proposed by the InterAction Council, 1 September 1997

Introductory Comment

It is time to talk about human responsibilities. Globalisation of the world economy is matched by global problems, and global problems demand global solutions on the basis of ideas, values and norms respected by all cultures and societies. Recognition of the equal and inalienable rights of all the people requires a foundation of freedom, justice and peace – but this also demands that rights and responsibilities be given equal importance to establish an ethical base so that all men and women can live peacefully together and fulfil their potential. A better social order both nationally and internationally cannot be achieved by laws, prescriptions and conventions alone, but needs a global ethic. Human aspirations for progress can only be realised by agreed values and standards applying to all people and institutions at all times. Next year will be the 50th anniversary of the Universal Declaration of Human Rights adopted by the UN. The anniversary would be an opportune time to adopt a Universal Declaration of Human Responsibilities, which would complement the Human Rights Declaration and strengthen it and help lead to a better world.

The following draft of human responsibilities seeks to bring freedom and responsibility into balance and to promote a move from the freedom of indifference to the freedom of involvement. If one person or government seeks to maximise freedom but does it at the expense of others, a larger number of people will suffer. If human beings maximise their freedom by plundering the natural resources of the earth, then future generations will suffer. The initiative to draft a Universal Declaration of Human Responsibilities is not only a way of balancing freedom with responsibility, but also a means of reconciling ideologies, beliefs and political views that were deemed antagonistic in the past. The proposed declaration points out that the exclusive insistence on rights can lead to endless dispute and conflict, that religious groups in pressing for their own freedom have a duty to respect the freedom of others. The basic premise should be to aim at the greatest amount of freedom possible, but also to develop the fullest sense of responsibility that will allow that freedom itself to grow. The InterAction Council has been working to draft a set of human ethical standards since 1987. But its work builds on the wisdom of religious leaders and sages down the ages who have warned that freedom without acceptance of responsibility can destroy the freedom itself, whereas when rights and responsibilities are balanced, then freedom is enhanced and a better world can be created.

The InterAction Council commends the following draft Declaration for your examination and support.

Preamble

Whereas recognition of the inherent dignity and of the equal and inalienable rights of all members of the human family is the foundation of freedom, justice and peace in the world and implies obligations or responsibilities, whereas the exclusive insistence on rights can result in conflict, division, and endless dispute, and the neglect of human responsibilities can lead to lawlessness and chaos, whereas the rule of law and the promotion of human rights depend on the readiness of men and women to act justly, whereas global problems demand global solutions which can only be achieved through ideas, values, and norms respected by all cultures and societies, whereas all people, to the best of their knowledge and ability, have a responsibility to foster a better social order, both at home and globally, a goal which cannot be achieved by laws, prescriptions, and conventions alone, whereas human aspirations for progress and improvement can only be realised by agreed values and standards applying to all people and institutions at all times,

Now, therefore, The General Assembly proclaims this Universal Declaration of Human Responsibilities as a common standard for all peoples and all nations, to the end that every individual and every organ of society, keeping this Declaration constantly in mind, shall contribute to the advancement of communities and to the enlightenment of all their members. We, the peoples of the world, thus renew and reinforce commitments already proclaimed in the Universal Declaration of Human Rights: namely, the full acceptance of the dignity of all people; their inalienable freedom and equality, and their solidarity with one another. Awareness and acceptance of these responsibilities should be taught and promoted throughout the world.

Fundamental Principles for Humanity

Article 1

Every person, regardless of gender, ethnic origin, social status, political opinion, language, age, nationality, or religion, has a responsibility to treat all people in a humane way.

Article 2

No person should lend support to any form of inhumane behavior, but all people have a responsibility to strive for the dignity and self-esteem of all others.

Article 3

No person, no group or organization, no state, no army or police stands above good and evil; all are subject to ethical standards. Everyone has a responsibility to promote good and to avoid evil in all things.

Article 4

All people, endowed with reason and conscience, must accept a responsibility to each and all, to families and communities, to races, nations, and religions in a spirit of solidarity: what you do not wish to be done to yourself, do not do to others.

Non-violence and Respect for Life

Article 5

Every person has a responsibility to respect life. No one has the right to injure, to torture or to kill another human person. This does not exclude the right of justified self-defence of individuals or communities.

Article 6

Disputes between states, groups or individuals should be resolved without violence. No government should tolerate or participate in acts of genocide or terrorism, nor should it abuse women, children, or any other civilians as instruments of war. Every citizen and public official has a responsibility to act in a peaceful, non-violent way.

Article 7

Every person is infinitely precious and must be protected unconditionally. The animals and the natural environment also demand protection. All people have a responsibility to protect the air, water and soil of the earth for the sake of present inhabitants and future generations.

Justice and Solidarity

Article 8

Every person has a responsibility to behave with integrity, honesty and fairness. No person or group should rob or arbitrarily deprive any other person or group of their property.

Article 9

All people, given the necessary tools, have a responsibility to make serious efforts to overcome poverty, malnutrition, ignorance, and inequality. They should promote sustainable development all over the world in order to assure dignity, freedom, security and justice for all people.

Article 10

All people have a responsibility to develop their talents through diligent endeavor; they should have equal access to education and to meaningful work. Everyone should lend support to the needy, the disadvantaged, the disabled and to the victims of discrimination.

Article 11

All property and wealth must be used responsibly in accordance with justice and for the advancement of the human race. Economic and political power must not be handled as an instrument of domination, but in the service of economic justice and of the social order.

Truthfulness and Tolerance

Article 12

Every person has a responsibility to speak and act truthfully. No one, however high or mighty, should speak lies. The right to privacy and to personal and professional confidentiality is to be respected. No one is obliged to tell all the truth to everyone all the time.

Article 13

No politicians, public servants, business leaders, scientists, writers or artists are exempt from general ethical standards, nor are physicians, lawyers and other professionals who have special duties to clients. Professional and other codes of ethics should reflect the priority of general standards such as those of truthfulness and fairness.

Article 14
The freedom of the media to inform the public and to criticize institutions of society and governmental actions, which is essential for a just society, must be used with responsibility and discretion. Freedom of the media carries a special responsibility for accurate and truthful reporting. Sensational reporting that degrades the human person or dignity must at all times be avoided.

Article 15
While religious freedom must be guaranteed, the representatives of religions have a special responsibility to avoid expressions of prejudice and acts of discrimination toward those of different beliefs. They should not incite or legitimize hatred, fanaticism and religious wars, but should foster tolerance and mutual respect between all people.

Mutual Respect and Partnership
Article 16
All men and all women have a responsibility to show respect to one another and understanding in their partnership. No one should subject another person to sexual exploitation or dependence. Rather, sexual partners should accept the responsibility of caring for each other's well-being.

Article 17
In all its cultural and religious varieties, marriage requires love, loyalty and forgiveness and should aim at guaranteeing security and mutual support.

Article 18
Sensible family planning is the responsibility of every couple. The relationship between parents and children should reflect mutual love, respect, appreciation and concern. No parents or other adults should exploit, abuse or maltreat children.

Conclusion
Article 19
Nothing in this Declaration may be interpreted as implying for any state, group or person any right to engage in any activity or to perform any act aimed at the destruction of any of the responsibilities, rights and freedom set forth in this Declaration and in the Universal Declaration of Human Rights of 1948.

CHAPTER 4

Towards Human Rights Ethics

Marrying Intuitionism, Reasoning and Communication

Cees J. Hamelink

Introduction

The central question of this chapter is how the basic principles of international human rights can contribute to the process of moral decision-making. We begin with arguing the significance of moral choice in the practice of health care and distinguish morality from ethics. This is followed by a presentation of the conventional methods of ethics and a critical analysis of these methods. Then we turn to the exploration of a human rights method of ethics. Crucial elements of this method are based upon the basic document of international human rights, the Universal Declaration of Human Rights. From this moral statement we extract both the way it portrays the human being and the basic standards of moral behaviour it proposes. In short, this leads to a method of ethics that combines intuitionism ("gut feelings") with rational justification (reasoned motivational arguments) and the individual personhood of the human being with social-communal embeddedness. The chapter concludes with exercises for the testing of the method of human rights ethics in practice.

Learning Objectives

After studying this chapter you will be able to:

- Understand the important role of intuition in moral choices
- Explain why moral choices need rational justification
- Discuss the shortcomings of conventional methods of ethics
- Explore a method of ethics that is based on human rights principles
- Test your capacity to justify moral choices in light of fundamental human rights standards

Health Care and Moral Choice

The practice of health care is a minefield of daily choices – not only clinical choices but also corporate and political choices that affect the quality of care and consequently

DOI: 10.4324/9781003408765-6

people's lives, their well-being, their self-esteem and self-confidence. Choices in health care range from end-of-life issues to problems of universal access to quality care or restrictive measures taken by governments during health crises. Often such choice-situations are presented as "moral dilemmas" although they may only partly address questions about morality. In most choice situations there are factual, conceptual and moral dimensions which need to be distinguished since the problems these dimensions pose need different solutions. In moral disputes it is not always differences of moral principle that are at stake: if we look closer we often discover that it is only a different interpretation of the facts or a different perspective that makes us disagree. Actually, the factual and conceptual dimensions of a situation cause sometimes more disagreement than the moral aspects! In many situations parties can agree on some common-sense moral principles, such as avoiding complicity with criminal regimes or the desire to protect people against the effects of toxic waste. However, the factual claim that choice A protects these principles more adequately than choice B may be fiercely contested. There are also choice situations in which we confront a conflict between basic moral premises we hold and other pressing interests, which can be of political, economic or personal nature. Even more complex are those situations that demand choices between two or more basic moral principles that are equally valid but demand different and conflicting courses of action. In such situations the physician, nurse, industrialist or politician can perform one of two (or more) actions but cannot do both (or all) of them. These situations produce real moral dilemmas since any course of action violates a fundamental moral value. If we violate principle A by doing X we commit a wrong. Equally, if we violate principle B by doing Y we commit a wrong. Dilemmas challenge us to choose between two or more wrongs. Choices may also be between moral principles and pressing personal or public interests.

The essential question is how to justify the choices that we make as moral. In making choices, we always face restrictive variables such as the available time, the complexity of the problem, contextual influences, different interpretations of factual factors and the limits of human cognitive capacity. These variables limit our rationality in decision-making. This phenomenon is often referred to as "bounded rationality", meaning that we tend to select choices that are satisfactory rather than optimal. In real-time decision-making we often cannot make a fully fledged cost-benefit analysis and have to make a decision that meets our "gut feelings" in a satisfactory way.

In reflecting on the perennial question "what is the right thing to do?" moral philosophers have asked over the centuries whether ethics can provide guidance in moral choice. Can ethical theory provide arguments that justify choice A versus choice B in specific situations?

Ethics and Morality

Dealing with moral choice requires ethics. We propose to understand ethics as the philosophical reflection on morality, immorality and a-morality in collective and individual human behaviour. Basic to the behaviour of human groups and individuals is a sense of "right" versus "wrong" that is inspired by a set of collective or individual values. Ethics is not a prescriptive exercise as morality is. Traditional morality may prohibit interventions such as abortion or euthanasia. Ethics reflects on such interventions in the light of moral values. It is descriptive, helps to understand moral choice and is primarily a learning exercise to fine-tune the process of moral choice. Ethics is the systematic reflection on the application of moral values to choices people make and on the accounting for the choices made. Morality refers to a set of deeply held, widely shared and relatively stable values within a community. Ethics as a philosophical enterprise involves the study of values and the justification for right and good actions, as represented by the classic works of Aristotle (virtue ethics), Kant (duty-based ethics) and Bentham and Mill (utilitarian and consequentialist ethics).

Moral Choice and Ethical Methods

Ethical theory seeks to introduce a degree of rationality and rigour into our moral deliberations. Our moral sentiments on any given topic will be less convincing to others if they are based on poor reasoning or factual inaccuracies. Moral philosophers will attempt to single out moral beliefs which are either self-contradictory or mutually exclusive. This is not to say that all our moral beliefs must be strictly rational but rather that our beliefs are better for being considered beliefs, rather than knee-jerk reactions to individual issues. There is also something to be said for the very process of theory-building. Sitting down to work out a coherent theory that explains our moral beliefs can illuminate existing contradictions and can help us to find patterns of moral thought that are more stable and that will be easier to learn and teach.

The Conventional Methods of Ethics

Conventional ethics can be divided into deontological (duty-based), consequentialist (effect-based) and virtue-based methods.

The Duty-based Method of Ethics

The duty-based approach, also called deontological ethics, is usually linked with the philosopher Immanuel Kant (1724–1804) who argued that moral acts stem from our duty to perform such acts. Kant coined the concept of the "categorical imperative" as the source for knowing what our duty is. The imperative instructs us to "Act only according to that maxim by which you can at the same time will that it should become a universal law". So, for example, lying is unethical because we could not universalise a maxim that said "One should always lie". Such a maxim would render all speech meaningless. We can, however, universalise the maxim, "Always speak truthfully", without running into a logical contradiction. We notice here that the duty-based approach says nothing about how easy or difficult it would be to carry out these maxims, only that it is our duty as rational creatures to do so. In acting according to a law that we have discovered to be rational according to our own universal reason, we are acting autonomously (in a self-regulating fashion) and thus are bound by duty, a duty we have given ourselves as rational creatures. We thus freely choose to bind ourselves to the moral law. For Kant, choosing to obey the universal moral law is the very nature of acting ethically.

Among duty-based approaches there is a distinction between act-based deontology and rule-based deontology. Act-based deontology is largely determined by the assumption that most people intuitively know how to choose in moral dilemmas. This implies that the crucial factor in moral choice is personal moral intuition. Professionals often claim that they instinctively know what the right thing to do is. Their moral feelings guide them flawlessly to responsible moral choices. The problem with this approach is the enormous latitude it offers for shady moral trickery which basically serves self-interest only. The method implies a large degree of arbitrariness, and moral arguments based upon intuition are difficult to justify, particularly when people use different definitions of what intuition is.

Rule-based deontology takes the position that rules based upon moral principles can provide guidance in moral choices. In essence, the method searches in concrete situations of moral choice for the moral rule that applies. For the professional practice, such rules may be articulated in a so-called code of conduct. However, given the great variety of choice situations and the inevitable general nature of the rules embedded in codes, these moral rules are not likely to provide concrete moral guidance. Moral prescriptions in codes suggest an almost universal applicability which is not realistic, since actors, situations and interests differ greatly over time and place. The rules of a code may prescribe that professionals should be truthful, but they will not explain how this general principle should be applied in concrete situations. Or the code may not tell its users when justifiable exceptions to its rules can and must be made. Also, the different rules in a code may conflict with each other, and the code does not explain how choices should be made when basic moral principles clash. A problem is also that no single moral rule has validity for all the different circumstances of its application in real life. Codes can be useful as instruments to identify an autonomous professional group. They provide a common set of rules for the members of a profession which contribute to the credibility and accountability of their professional performance. A code of conduct tells the clients of professionals what quality they may expect from the professional conduct. Although codes of conduct can certainly provide a starting point for ethical enquiry and debate, they fail to provide concrete moral guidance. Most importantly, codes offer a set of guidelines usually in a unilateral way to the professional group involved, medical doctors, lawyers, notaries, social workers or journalists. This is odd since professions usually imply relationships between professionals and clients. In most professional codes there are provisions that deal with this relationship. Professionals are expected to respect the autonomy of their clients, to avoid abuse of the vulnerable position of the client, to fully and honestly inform the client, to maintain the confidentiality of the communication and to act with expertise and carefulness. All this attention paid to the client is, however, still a rather one-sided approach to the relationship. It would seem more accurate to perceive the professional-client relation as an interactive process which depends upon a mutual commitment. This implies that also the client/patient actively contributes to the professional performance and has both rights and responsibilities. If one accepts the interactive character of the professional-client relationship, it follows that professional ethics cannot be limited to the rights and wrongs of the professionals only and should also be ethics for their clients. The case for this interactive ethics can be defended by demonstrating that all parties involved face moral choices in connection with health care.

What is actually needed then is a covenant upon which the parties involved agree. It would seem more useful for the protection of patients' interests to have an agreed-upon compact of rights and responsibilities between medical experts and their clients than a set of moral guidelines for the doctors only. The – often debated – limited capacity for the enforcement of a code of conduct is obviously related not only to its voluntary nature but also to its unilateral scope. A party concludes a contract with itself and judges the validity and applicability of the terms of the contract unilaterally. A contract between more parties becomes a different matter altogether. Parties can appeal to a common commitment to honour certain rules and could eventually ask outsiders (courts, mediators) to arbitrate. It could well be that a covenant between parties provides – if not always the perfect guidance in choice making – at least a common framework for the ethical reflection. The gravest problem, however, with deontological methods is their neglect of the consequences of moral choices. This does create a peculiar tension when codes of conduct are used. The rules in codes suggest that those who use the code will act in responsible ways. However, since the code prescribes conduct in accordance with its general rules and principles, this does not necessarily imply a responsible attitude towards the consequences of such conduct.

Summary

Duty-based methods focus on the duties and obligations that we have in a given situation and consider what moral obligations we have and what things we should never do. Moral conduct is defined by doing one's duties and doing the right thing, and the goal is performing the correct action. This framework has the advantage of creating a system of rules that has consistent expectations of all people; if an action is morally correct or a duty is required, it would apply to every person in a given situation. This even-handedness encourages treating everyone with equal dignity and respect. This framework also focuses on following moral rules or duties regardless of the outcome and thus allows for the possibility that one might have acted morally, even if there is a bad result. It might require actions which are known to produce harms, even though they are strictly in keeping with a particular moral rule. It also does not provide for a way to determine which duty we should follow if we are presented with a situation in which two or more duties conflict. It can also be rigid in applying the notion of duty to everyone regardless of personal situation and does not in any convincing manner address situations of basic conflicts among equally valid duties. Deontology provides no answer in the case that fundamental values or obligations collide. It also does not assist us in determining which is the lesser wrong in a moral dilemma. The duty-based method fails to take into account other variables (such as pressing interests or consequences) and is therefore not helpful in real-life choices between principles and interests.

The Effects-based or Utilitarian Method of Ethics

This method goes back to the Greek philosopher Epicurus of Samos (341–270 BC), who argued that the best life is the life with the least pain. Inspired by this, the British philosopher Jeremy Bentham (1748–1832) designed a system in which acts could be described as good or bad depending upon the level of pleasure or pain they would produce. John Stuart Mill (1806–1873), who was a student of Bentham, changed the standard for the good life from pleasure to happiness. This method requires that in moral choice-making good versus bad consequences be weighed. These effects may concern individual self-interest or the best for all people.

The Consequentialist Method Can Be Divided in Act-based Utilitarianism and Rule-based Utilitarianism

Act-based utilitarianism is casuistic, meaning that from case to case it must be considered what type of conduct has the best consequences. This casuistry is necessary since general rules and principles are of little use in the great variety of choice situations that real life confronts us with. However attractive this may seem, the approach has certain drawbacks. First, who defines what optimal consequences of certain choices are? Second, it is extremely difficult to establish what optimal consequences are under different conditions for different actors.

Rule-utilitarianism assumes that one finds sufficient similarity between choice situations for general rules to be useful. In this sense this method resembles rule-based deontology. Both methods propose that general rules should define what moral acts are. However, because of the large variety of real choice situations, rule-based utilitarianism is bound to fail. Moreover – as in the case of act-utilitarianism – there is no unequivocal understanding of what constitutes the best consequence (effect) for the largest number of people.

An important attraction of utilitarian methods is that they take the consequences of moral choices seriously. A complex problem, however, is that most of the time people cannot know the consequences of their actions. Moreover, consequentialist type method implies the risk that beneficial ends justify immoral means. In the professional practice, the optimal consequences of moral decision-making are often identified as the effects that serve the "common good". This suggests a societal consensus about the notion of "common good". In reality, this is a highly evasive concept that has many different interpretations. In all societies, opinions about what constitutes the "common good" are divided. Actually, its meaning is often defined by the most powerful groups in society and rarely coincides with the needs of the less powerful. Henry Sidgwick's (1838–1900) moral philosophy provides a rational and systematic approach to ethics, based on the principle of the greatest happiness for the greatest number. While his utilitarian approach has been influential, it has also been subject to criticism and debate. Nevertheless, Sidgwick's work continues to be an important influence on the development of ethical thought and the study of morality.

Effect-based approaches focus on the future effects of possible courses of action, considering the people who will be directly or indirectly affected. We ask what outcomes are desirable in a given situation and consider moral conduct to be whatever will achieve the best consequences. The person using the consequentialist frame wants to produce the most good. Among the advantages of this ethical method is that focusing on the results of an action is a pragmatic approach. It helps in situations involving many people, some of whom may benefit from the action, while others may not. On the other hand, it is not always possible to predict the consequences of an action, so some actions that are expected to produce good consequences might actually end up harming people. Additionally, people sometimes react negatively to the use of compromise which is an inherent part of this approach, and they recoil from the implication that the end justifies the means. It also does not include a pronouncement that certain things are always wrong, as even the most heinous actions may result in a good outcome for some people, and this framework allows for these actions to then be moral. The consequentialist method does not inform us of how to establish what optimal consequences are under different circumstances for different actors. Consequentialism also poses the problem that most of the time we cannot know the consequences of our actions. Apart from the difficulty that in a consequentialist method beneficial ends may justify immoral means, we get no guidance in resolving hard moral choices.

The Virtue-based Method of Ethics

For the Greek philosopher Aristotle (384BC–322 BC), ethics was a practical enterprise. Its aim was to promote human happiness. He writes several times "that the purpose of lecturer and student is not merely to learn the truth, but to improve men and make them happier" (Allan, 1970, p. 125). In Aristotelian ethics the "telos" is happiness or well-being, and this is "the ultimate standard of reference for all our moral judgments" (ibidem, 126). Necessary for human happiness are two intellectual virtues: "sophia" (theoretical wisdom) and "phronesis" (practical wisdom). Aristotle argues that practical wisdom is crucial for "moral virtue" since without the discipline of emotions moral virtue would be blind. In the recent rise of attention to virtue ethics, Alasdair MacIntyre (1981) plays a key role. In his view the key question is how to make moral choices that lead to living a good life. The judgment about which choices we should make to achieve this "telos" depends upon good character. In a way, MacIntyre re-writes the Aristotelian view of an ethical teleology. In the Aristotelian sense, virtue ethics emphasises the wholeness of people's lives and is less concerned with the specific acts that people may perform in certain situations. MacIntyre emphasises the importance of realising the standards of excellence that are definitive for cooperative human activity (MacIntyre, 1981, p. 175) rather than focusing on practice-independent obligations of a moral agent (deontological ethics) or the consequences of particular actions (utilitarianism).

Summary

The key question in the virtue frame is "Am I a virtuous person?" In the virtue-based method of ethics, we try to identify the character traits (either positive or negative) that might motivate us in a given situation. We are concerned with what kind of person we should be and what our actions indicate about our character. We define moral behaviour as whatever a virtuous person would do in the situation, and we seek to develop similar virtues. Obviously, this framework is useful in situations that ask what sort of person one should be. As a way of making sense of the world, it allows for a wide range of behaviours to be called moral, as there might be many different types of good character and many paths to developing it. Consequently, it takes into account all parts of human experience and their role in ethical deliberation, as it believes that all of one's experiences, emotions and thoughts can influence the development of one's character. Although this framework takes into account a variety of human experiences, it also makes it difficult to resolve disputes, as there can often be considerable disagreement about virtuous traits. Also, because the framework looks at character, it is not particularly good at helping someone to decide what actions to take in a given situation or to determine the rules that would guide one's actions. Also, because it emphasises the importance of role models and education to moral behaviour, it can sometimes merely reinforce current cultural norms as the standard of moral behaviour.

Critique and Additions: Context, Dialogue and Intuition

Context-based Approach

The application of conventional ethical methods of deontological, utilitarian or virtue-ethics signature provides little or no help in the resolution of concrete moral dilemmas in real-life situations. Moral principles – in difficult choice situations – do not provide guidance for unequivocal, consensual decisions. Examples can be found in choices about euthanasia, abortion, suicide, armed conflict, social security, immigration and drug policy. Concrete experiences in such fields as medical and business ethics have led "to a serious if not widespread erosion of confidence in the power of normative theory to decisively guide the resolution of real practical problems" (Winkler & Coombs, 1993, p. 3). In the quest for a more adequate approach it has been proposed to conceive of morality as "an evolving social instrument" that is part of a specific cultural context (Winkler & Coombs, 1993, p. 3). This suggests a contextual approach to moral decision-making which

> adopts the general idea that moral problems must be resolved within the interpretive complexities of concrete circumstances, by appeal to relevant historical and cultural traditions, with reference to critical institutional and professional norms and virtues, and by relying primarily upon the method of comparative case analysis.
> *(Winkler & Coombs, 1993, p. 4)*

The contextualist approach rejects the deductive model of moral problem-solving and prefers an inductive model of moral argument. From the contextualist perspective, a primary task in situations of choice is the precise interpretation of the moral issue at stake. The first step is the attempt to understand in detail what the basic choice is in a concrete case. This differs from the deductive approach where one begins with a general moral theory or with general moral principles and applies these to the concrete case. The contextualist approach proposes a comparative case analysis through which resolutions to new choices are sought by reasoning from solutions that were preferred in similar situations. In the course of the inductive moral argument, questions are asked about the institutional and cultural settings that were preferred in similar situations. In this light, questions are also asked about the consequences of choice and the interests involved: "where does the choice lead to?" and "Is this desirable?" "How are benefits versus damages of choice distributed?" And "Whose interests are served with a particular choice?" Who gains and who loses? Contextualism offers the possibility of a more eclectic model in which the ethical dialogue moves back and forth between general moral principles and specific details of choice-situations. This dialogical type of ethics views the resolution of moral choice-situations as a mutual learning experience. It is a process in which people learn from each other, listen to the outsider and try to understand the rationale of the outsider. In the ethical dialogue, people also discover that the moral practices of "us" are not always morally defensible and that those by "them" are not always morally despicable. The ethical dialogue must be conceived as a reiterative and dynamic process since health care situations and medical practices change over time and space.

Discursive Approach

The deductive approach to moral choice is increasingly problematic as modern societies become more democratic, pluralistic and multicultural. Moral standards cannot any longer be authoritatively imposed upon all members of such societies. Under these conditions ethics can evolve in a legitimate fashion only through the dialogue among all those concerned. As German social philosopher Jurgen Habermas proposes, moral standards are valid only when all those concerned would give their consent following their common deliberations (Habermas, 1993, p. 66). Herewith the basis is given of what has been termed a communicative or discursive ethics (Apel, 1988). In the dialogue it is explored upon which "minima moralia" societies can find basic and common agreement. Since there are never ideal solutions for moral choices and since any moral choice is essentially contestable, the ethical dialogue does not automatically lead to the only acceptable moral choice but renders moral choices communicative acts that are transparent for all those affected by them. The proposal for an ethical dialogue assumes there are always various plausible solutions to morality regarding the choice situations. Therefore, ethical reflection should not focus on identifying the single correct solution but should rather concentrate on the due process of the moral argumentation. The ethical dialogue does not depart from a consensus on fundamental principles and moral values but seeks those solutions to moral dispute that optimally accommodate the parties' interests and principles.

Intuition-based Approach

In discursive ethics, moral judgement is reached by rational reasoning and consensual argumentation (Apel and Habermas). Different from this is an approach to moral choice that takes our intuitive judgments very seriously. This approach is theoretically best embedded in the intuitionist model of Jonathan Haidt (2001). The basic claims about moral positions in this model are that intuitions come first and that they are justified or explained after the fact in order to convince others of the legitimacy of our moral decision. The model de-emphasises the role of reasoning in reaching moral conclusions. Haidt asserts that moral judgment is primarily moved by intuition, with reasoning playing a smaller role in most of our moral decision-making. Conscious thought processes serve as a kind of post-hoc justification of our decisions. Haidt's model also states that moral reasoning is more likely to be interpersonal than private, reflecting on social motives (such as reputation or alliance-building) rather than on abstract principles. The model proposes that social and cultural factors are more important in moral decision-making than individual rational reasoning. It is important that Haidt's social intuitionist model (SIM) stresses the role of social interaction in moral judgments.

Moral intuitionism is already in 19th century moral philosophy discussed by, among others, Henry Sidgwick (1838–1900) under the heading of "Common Sense Morality". This is a utilitarian approach that takes seriously the intuitions that evolved in the human evolutionary process and that point to the common sense of promoting general happiness. Sidgwick, however, adds that "without being disposed to deny that conduct commonly to be judged right is so, we may yet require some deeper explanation why it is so" (Sidgwick, 1981, p. 102). This means that, although accepting that the morality of common sense is sound, we may still attempt "to find for it a philosophical basis . . . and to get one or more principles more absolutely and undeniably true and evident, from which the current rules might be deduced" (ibidem, 102).

A fundamental critique of the conventional methods of ethics – Kantian deontology and Benthamite consequentialism – is their mechanistic format. They offer engineering models for moral choice. But do people make moral choices like engineers build bridges? The engineer has a goal – a solid bridge, the best possible bridge, a happy bridge – and chooses what according to engineering knowledge is the best method to achieve the preferred bridge. The engineer practices a craft. As life is more art than craft, we should ask whether moral decision-making should not be more an art than an engineering craft. The prevailing methods of ethics seem to prefer the engineering method that proposes "how to do it" manuals with instruction of how to apply formal rules (about duties or consequences) to concrete problems. However, the manual does not help us to solve the most basic question of "why be moral?" In ethics as craft we have a "telos" and work towards the achievement of that goal. The goal may be happiness or well-being. But, is daily life really about pursuing happiness or well-being? In reality we may not pursue happiness but try to make life meaningful. We try to make something out of life. As artists we do not know what the end product will be. As Ronald Duska phrases it, "The true artist does not know his end: he discovers it as he works it out" (Duska in Sommers & Sommers, 1989, p. 560).

Although international human rights lean towards the temptation to define a "telos" with the instruction to apply principles and codified rights to achieve this goal, the human rights vision on the human being enables a non-formal, creative exercise in moral choice that is more art than craft. This vision is not mechanistic as in the moral theories of Immanuel Kant or Jeremy Bentham where moral acting follows rational procedures. The basic vision of the human being is a holistic one. Human beings act morally as a "whole" which is in a combination of rational and irrational faculties.

Human Rights Ethics: Intuition and Reason, Personhood and Community

In search of a method of ethics that can guide moral decision-making in the health care practice, we propose to explore a human rights-based approach. This leads us to an ethics as basic reflection on human rights morality that is based upon the portrayal of the human being in human rights documents. The human rights method of ethics deviates from conventional, largely engineering, approaches to moral choice-making. It is more an art than a craft. This means that the process of choice is not a mechanistic procedure but comes closer to the way people – in daily practice – make moral choices. This approach in which "making the best of it" does not ignore obligations, principles and goals but gives them a more modest place in human realities. This way there is more space for holistic thinking, creativity and intuition. Basic to this method is a communal process of deliberation, reflection and evaluation in which the quality of caring is –iteratively questioned. Care-givers and care-receivers alike engage with the question of mutual understanding. In the search for genuine caring, the main driver is the human rights vision of the human being in search of self-realisation as being with others. The human rights perspective is that we are "humans in making". We are part of a process of self-realisation in relation to others. We discover who we are in a communicative community with others who are different from us. Personal identity is found in the encounter with alterity. In the encounter human persons can make the transition from what they are to what they can be. In this transition the environmental context is always in flux. It is like a river that is never the same and we cannot foresee where our lives may take us. We play with the cards that were handed out to us and there is no guarantee that the best cards will yield the best result.

No method of ethics guarantees that the choices we make are the best. The choices that are best according to the engineering method can work out in a fatal way. Most of our choice-making is acting in uncertainty. The method of human rights ethics deals with this by accepting that there is not always a satisfactory rational justification of moral choices. There can only be a collective conclusion that we made the best out of the situation as free and autonomous persons.

Intuition and Reason

Our search for a human rights method of ethics is inspired by moral philosopher Henry Sidgwick when he writes

> Probably most moral men believe that their moral sense or instinct in any case will guide them fairly right, but also that there are general rules for determining rights action in different department of conduct; and that it is possible to find a philosophical explanation, by which they may be deduced from a smaller number of fundamental principles.
>
> *(1981, p. 103)*

In human moral evolution, humans acquired the capacity to intuitively judge what is good for all but also the capacity to reason why this is so. The Universal Declaration of Human Rights (UDHR) opens with an intuitive statement that is not rationally argued. As the 1776 USA Declaration of Independence states when it refers to equality, liberty and the pursuit of happiness, "We hold these truths to be self-evident", the UDHR accepts the moral intuitionism that proposes that moral judgment is primarily moved by intuition. The UDHR departs from a common-sense morality that is not the result of inferential reasoning from some moral belief. However, in its Article 1, the Declaration also states that the human being is endowed with reason and conscience. This means we are capable of rational justification of our decisions. As intuitions may be inconsistent, dubitable and based upon misleading beliefs, they need justification on reasonable grounds. We propose that in the justification process the guiding principles play a crucial role. These principles of dignity, freedom, equality and security will be discussed later in this book. The implication of their significant role in the justification process is a plea for human rights education as it may be expected that the fundamental normative standards of human rights over time become a natural element in our moral decision-making. The challenge of the human rights method of ethics is to find a balance between intuitionist common sense morality and a process of justificatory reasoning about moral decisions.

Gigerenzer in his book *Gut Feelings* (2007) pleads for the development of a science of intuitive decision-making and for the training of medical professionals to expertly apply this method. As medical intuitions are a reality, we may be well advised to improve and fine-tune them, as intuitions are based upon moral principles but without us being aware of them. A beginning of the fine-tuning process is becoming aware of the principles or rules on which moral choices are based.

Summary

Intuitive judgments have a valid place in moral choice-making and from a human rights perspective should be taken seriously. We can fine-tune intuitive judgments by empathising with other people's realities and by engaging with people of different beliefs and convictions. Intuitions may conflict with others we hold with equal conviction. Sometimes intuitions cannot be reconciled. There may be a diversity of moral intuitions, and people do often doubt and even repudiate certain intuitions, and the evident origin of some intuitions in social prejudice or self-interest makes it untenable to suppose that intuitions are infallible apprehensions of moral reality by some special faculty of moral perception. Since intuitions may dubitable and inconsistent, they need justification on reasonable grounds; which is they need arguments based upon historical knowledge and/or social and psychological empirical experience. People tend to trust their own intuitions and mistrust those of others. Having made a choice based upon our intuitive judgment of what was the correct thing to do is helpful in understanding what we did – to reason with ourselves and others involved why this choice made sense. This is a retrospective rationalisation of what we did. Questions to address are "did my choice make sense to me?", "why did it make sense?" and "did my choice make sense to others affected by my choice?"

From the sense-making exercise, a next step would be to explore and become aware of the moral rules and principles on which the intuitive judgment was based. Since we are in search of human rights-based health care, it makes sense to test these judgments against the key moral principles of international human rights. This is a process of rational reasoning that also subjects these key principles to critical reflection. The assumption underlying this exercise is that the credibility of the intuitive judgment is enhanced if it can be subsumed under moral principle that has independent credibility. In this textbook we have chosen as moral framework the basic moral principles of the International Human Rights Regime. These principles find their justification in their historical origins and their status in international law, in common law and in universally shared moral values. As the justification process is an exercise in critical thinking, human rights principles themselves also have to be critically questioned by testing their consistency with other moral beliefs.

Person and Community

The UDHR comes from a liberal individualist tradition, but the drafters were aware that we are as members of societies communal beings. Whereas conventional methods of ethics entertain a conception of morality that is largely an individualistic, human rights ethics takes into account that people are part of a larger environment. Morality is linked with our membership in historical communities. The morality of international human rights recognises the importance of community and social connections. The "everyone" in the articles of the UDHR are members of a society. This emphasis on community and social support reflects an image of the human being as an individual who thrives in a supportive and inclusive environment. The justification of moral choice is sought in an argumentation community (Thys, 1989, p. 68). The validity of our moral choices needs to be tested in the communitarian dialogue. Therefore, the choice made is not merely an atomistic event; it is made by persons belonging to a community and thus needs reflection in the primary community. In a hospital setting, for example, this is the community of patients, nurses, physicians and managers.

In the human rights perspective, the human being is gifted with communicative capacity. Therefore, the justification process is a communal and communicative process guided by human rights standards. Moral choice from a human rights perspective is a process of social interaction that is iterative and creative: more art than craft. It is characterised by care, intuition and passion. Human rights ethics is a process of social interaction and as a communicative process, a communication process – a deep dialogue – within the network of all those directly involved. The careful reasoning in the dialogue can lead to agreement on moral choice or to a clarification on why people disagree. The communal dialogue concludes with these questions: did the process make sense? What did we learn from it?

The key requirements of a deep dialogue are trust, patience and freedom. It is essential that this process itself meets the human rights standards for communicative processes. These are communicative dignity, communicative freedom, communicative equality and communicative security.

- Communicative dignity means that human behaviour avoids the humiliation of persons through de-individualisation, discrimination, disempowerment and degrading.
- Communicative freedom means that people are free to accept or reject each other's claims on the basis of reasons they can evaluate.
- Communicative equality means that in communicative behaviour the participants are equal to initiate communication, that speech acts are symmetrical, and that communication roles are reciprocal.
- Communicative security means communicating in a caring manner. Security means knowing you will be cared for. A secure society is a community of mutual care in which people are protected against forms of verbal and non-verbal harm to their physical, mental or moral integrity.

This communication process is a deep dialogue as "the speech of genuine conversation in which men understand one another and come to a mutual understanding" (Buber, 1999, p. 236). This conversation requires trust which means that I need to know that what the other says is genuine and the other should be assured that what I say is authentic. In the authentic conversation you expect that the other accepts your word as genuine (Buber, 1999, p. 238) "for I can only speak to someone in the true sense of the term if I expect him to accept my word as genuine". Communicative authenticity also means the challenge to say "I do not know". Most of us live in professional or personal worlds where this poses a big problem as we are expected as academics or parents to have answers to problems. Communicative authenticity implies that we feel free to speak up. This means that we have to overcome an almost natural inclination towards self-censorship that makes us not say things we wanted to say because we are afraid of the consequences. By leaving out the issues of conflict, we may reach superficial public agreement, but in fact we cause deep fractures. We often create a common comfortable discourse and leave out what we really should say, desire, hope for, expect or fear. Genuine communication, however, implies that people do not just talk to others but talk with each other and in this interaction feel free to say what they think and thus speak up.

Participation in deep dialogues is an engagement with a very difficult mode of human communication. It requires the skills to question one's own judgments and assumptions, to reflectively and actively listen and to be silent. Caught up in our own prejudices, fears and feelings, we often listen to ourselves and not to others. We often accuse the other of not listening and of being prejudiced and prefer to not see those flaws in our own thinking. We seldom ask real questions and more often than not produce opinionated statements to which we add a question mark. In many encounters that are termed dialogue, the participants do not question their own assumptions and take positions that they see as non-negotiable. We all bring assumptions about ourselves, others, the world, our societies, relationships and ways of life to the encounter. We tend to hold our assumptions to be truths and defend them even against overwhelming evidence of their flaws. The critical core of this "deep" dialogue is formed by the art of asking real questions and the art listening! These arts are not necessarily part of the human mental constitution. The authentic conversation is slow and needs time for ideas to sink in and to understand perspectives different from our own. This requires patience, a formidable challenge in times when many providers and recipients of health care are in permanently a hurry to diagnose, to treat, to cure and to receive clinical results and effective therapies. In this frenzied process, engaging in genuine conversation may seem a waste of time. However, for the deep dialogue we need to learn the willingness and the openness to "waste time" or, in Bertrand Russell's words, to praise idleness (Russell, 1935).

Guidelines for the Ethical Deep Dialogue
On the Inter-personal Level
A good start of the ethical dialogue is the internal dialogue: a conversation we have with ourselves. This dialogue is not just a monologue, as it often involves multiple dimensions of our identity. In this conversation we may critically question ourselves or encourage and support ourselves.

In this internal dialogue you may ask:

- Was the choice I made based upon "gut feelings"?
- Can I make these feelings explicit?
- Can I trace by which values, interests, emotions and experiences my intuitive choice was motivated?
- Where do these motivations come from: parents, other family members, schoolteachers, religious leaders, professional role-models?
- How does my intuitive choice relate to such basic human rights principles as freedom, dignity, equality and security?

For the dialogue with colleagues/peer/friends the process can be:

- Telling your story and explaining which choices you faced and what choice you made
- If possible, telling the story also from the perspective of the patient: he/she tells why the request for a choice was important. Hearing from the patient why the choice you made was good or bad
- Talking with the group about which personal interests or institutional interests were served or disserved by choice A versus an alternative choice
- Questioning whether these interests can be justified by non-subjective and non-intuitive arguments
- Discussing whether your preferred choice was more or less in line with generally adopted professional rules and institutional codes of practice
- Identifying for which actors your preferred choice has (or may have) important consequences and questioning whether these consequences can be rationally justified

- Discussing whether the consequences of your choice could be reasonably foreseen
- Discussing whether any harm was done to those involved
- Could this possible harm have been avoided or minimised?
- Discussing with the group how strong your arguments for the rejection of an alternative choice are
- Talking about what would have been your choice if the roles had been reversed and the choice affected you
- Exploring whether you are ready to account publicly for your choice
- Rating your choice against such basic human rights principles as: respect for dignity, autonomy and security of the others involved. Discussing this rating in the group

On the Institutional Level

Not only does the work floor makes choices, but choices are also made on the level of institutional governance that have human rights implications. Let us take a hospital that aspires to profile itself as providing human rights-based health care. The institution has to make a decision, for example on the security of its data systems and the use of artificial intelligence in managing these systems. Sometimes the institution has to reflect on the human rights quality of its past decisions. This requires an openness for retrospective assessment and a readiness to learn from mistakes. As institutional choices may have important implications for the future, they need a form of prospective assessment of possible outcomes. This dialogue may focus on the question of how to avoid violations of human rights principles but also on how to make choices that promote and protect such principles. As the human rights method suggests, those responsible for the management and governance of health care institutions should try to find a rational justification for institutional choices in the light of the question of how they relate to human rights principles. This means that in both retrospective and prospective assessments it is important to realise that there will always be alternative options for achieving the objective of optimal human rights-based health care. The institutional choices (made or to be made) may or may not lead to the attainment of the objective. There may be positive versus negative outcomes and from these outcomes events may emerge that are expected or unexpected and the effects of which may be desirable or undesirable. Also among parties affected by the choice are the medical staff, the patients and the insurance companies, and there may be consensus or dissent on these effects. The key question in this complicated choice process is how institutional choices relate to the human rights framework. As future outcomes of institutional choices may be uncertain, it is crucial to reflect on past decisions and let their human rights assessment guide them to an optimisation of choices still to be made.

In addition to hospital level decision-making or other meso-level institutions, human rights ethics can also contribute to making just decisions at national and/or international levels.

Concluding Remarks

The method of human rights ethics stresses that moral decision-making is an iterative process in which participants learn to get better at fine-tuning their choices. Crucial elements of the human rights method of ethics are based upon the UDHR. This basic human rights document portrays the human being as an individual embedded in communal life with a unique capacity for compassionate communication. Human rights inspire a method of ethics that combines "gut feelings" with rational justifications of arguments in processes of moral choice. It is important to see that this does not imply an opposition between intuition and rationality. Intuitions have a rational cognitive dimension that helps us to know the world around us. They also have a strategic rationality that helps us to act in the world (Scarantino & De Sousa, 2021). What is crucial is that moral choices will always have be accounted for in a genuine conversation among those involved in or affected by the choices we make. The key elements of the justification of moral choice are the essential normative principles of the international human rights framework.

Questions for Discussion

- What was an important choice you made based upon "gut feelings"?
- Can you make these feelings explicit and trace their sources?
- Did your intuitive choices relate to basic human rights principles?
- Can you think of an institutional choice where human rights ethics may be a helpful tool?
- Can you think of policy choice on the national level where human rights ethics may be a helpful tool?

References

Allan, D. J. (1970). *The philosophy of Aristotle*. Oxford University Press.

Apel, K. O. (1988). *Diskurs und Verantwortung*. Suhrkamp.

Buber, M. (1999). *Pointing the way: Collected essays*. Humanity Books.

Duska, R. (1989). Literature and moral education. In C. Sommers & F. Sommers (Eds.), *Vice & virtue in everyday life* (pp. 553–566). Harcourt Brace.

Gigerenzer, G. (2007). *Gut feelings*. Viking Press.

Habermas, J. (1993). *Moral consciousness and communicative action*. MIT Press.

Haidt, J. (2001). The emotional dog and its rational tail: A social intuitionist approach to moral judgment. *Psychological Review, 108*(4), 814–834.

Russell, B. (1935). *In praise of idleness* (1996 ed.). Routledge.

Sidgwick, H. (1981). *The methods of ethics* (7th ed. of 1907). Hackett Publishing Company.

Thys, W. (1989). *De deugd weer in het midden*. Uitgeverij Pelckmans.

Winkler, E. R., & Coombs, J. R. (Eds.). (1993). *Applied ethics*. Basil Blackwell.

For Further Reading

Fiurna, G. C. (1995). *The other side of language: A philosophy of listening*. Routledge.

Gewirth, A. (1981). *Reason and morality*. The University of Chicago Press.

Hamelink, C. J. (1988). *The technology gamble: A study of technology choice*. Ablex Publishing.

MacIntyre, A. (1981). *After virtue*. University of Notre Dame Press.

Morsink, J. (1990). *The UDHR*. University of Pennsylvania Press.

Nino, C. S. (1991). *The ethics of human rights*. Oxford University Press.

Parks, E. S. (2019). *The ethics of listening*. Lexington Books.

Raz, J. (1994). *Ethics in the public domain*. Clarendon Press.

Sandel, M. J. (1982). *Liberalism and the limits of justice*. Cambridge University Press.

Scarantino, A., & de Sousa, R. (2021). Chapter 10: Rationality and emotions. In E. N. Zalta (Ed.), *The Stanford encyclopedia of philosophy*. Stanford University Press.

Walzer, M. (1983). *Spheres of justice: A defense of pluralism and equality*. Basic Books.

Health and Human Rights of Othered and Marginalised Groups

Part II of the textbook explores the complexities of health inequities and human rights violations experienced by groups that are "othered" and marginalised across the globe. Despite the presence of the international human rights framework, including declarations, treaties and conventions as introduced in Part I of this book, important gaps remain in the implementation and enforcement of commitments to autonomy, dignity, equality and security in health. Part II adopts a thematic approach to introduce and explore some of the key compounded challenges faced by particular "othered" individuals or groups in achieving their human rights and human right to health.

"Othering" is a concept that refers to the process of perceiving or portraying someone, a group, a community or even a country or a region as fundamentally different or alien, often leading to marginalisation and exclusion (Brons, 2015). This concept is rooted in existentialist and post-colonial thought. Simone de Beauvoir made a significant contribution through her feminist philosophical work, particularly in *The Second Sex* (1949). In this book, she explores how women have historically been considered and treated as the "Other", resulting in an inferior position in relation to men, who are considered the default or the norm. Othering also has roots in post-colonial theory; in Edward Said's seminal work *Orientalism* (1978) he explores how the West constructs the East as the "Other" in order to define itself. Given that othering involves perceiving or portraying individuals or groups as fundamentally different or alien, this sets groups up in unequal opposition based on certain characteristics. This implicit hierarchy establishes a sense of superiority versus inferiority, bolstering the identity and status of one individual, group or even country or region, while marginalising others. Othering operates by distancing and stigmatising those perceived as different, alien or "Other", thereby reinforcing existing social structures (Brons, 2015).

The concept has since evolved through the contributions of theorists across disciplines such as sociology, anthropology and feminist theory. Its significance in global health lies in its ability to shed light on the intricate connections between health inequities and processes of marginalisation. The UDHR is founded on the principle that

DOI: 10.4324/9781003408765-7

human rights are inherent to all individuals by virtue of their humanity. However, when individuals or groups are relegated to the status of the "Other", their humanity is undermined, consequently eroding the universality of human rights. This process of othering has historically led to and continues to cause significant health disparities among marginalised groups. Such violations stem from deep-seated (cultural) beliefs, attitudes and behaviours that perpetuate this inferior status.

In six chapters, Part II of the book explores such challenges for various individuals, groups and communities in the context of human rights. For instance, girls and women seeking reproductive health services might encounter compounded stigmatisation and barriers to accessing health services, such as abortion services. Individuals with mental health conditions can be subjected to coercive treatments or denied their autonomy. Indigenous peoples may face discrimination due to violations of self-determination and cultural misunderstanding in health and beyond. This part of the book explores how human rights violations are not simply infringements on the integrity of individuals who happen to belong to certain groups. Rather, they originate from deeply rooted beliefs, attitudes and behaviours, in the context of systems of privilege and oppression, that perpetuate the inferior status of these groups and superior status of others, ultimately undermining the right to the "highest attainable standard of health".

References

Brons, L. L. (2015). Othering, an analysis. *Transcience, 6*.
de Beauvoir, S. (2010). *The second sex*. Vintage Books.
Said, E. W. (1978). *Orientalism*. Pantheon Books.

CHAPTER 5

Sexual and Reproductive Health and Rights

A Perspective on Gender Bias and Stereotyping in Health

Marlies J. Visser

Introduction

This chapter comprises two sections, each exploring critical aspects of sexual and reproductive health in the context of human rights. The first section serves as an introduction to sexual and reproductive health and their position in the human rights framework, examining this rights area against the backdrop of the intricate and compounded challenges to attain the "highest attainable standard of health", especially for women and girls. This section introduces the multiple dimensions of sexual and reproductive rights (SRHR) and their centrality in health, well-being and human rights. Additionally, this section discusses the evolving conceptualisations of SRHR within the context of human rights and explores its interconnectedness with other human rights standards and principles.

The second part of the chapter shifts focus to (the impact of) societal perceptions on women and girls, shaped by their position as the "other". Gender systems[1] and hierarchies have entrenched themselves within our health systems and research, influencing access to and quality of health care services. This section discusses various ways gender stereotypes and stigmatisation can perpetuate health inequities and undermine human rights within sexual and reproductive health. The section highlights the inextricable link among gender, stigma and health and argues for urgency of considering compounded forms of stigma and discrimination as violations of human rights. Such violations require urgent attention in medical and health research and care. Lastly, this chapter presents a case study highlighting the pivotal role of women's organisations in safeguarding the right to safe abortion services including a statement for discussion for readers to develop and reflect on their own position in regard to abortion services.

A comprehensive understanding of the progress made and challenges in ensuring the highest attainable standard of sexual and reproductive health is indispensable to grasp the intricate ways in which individuals, especially women and girls, experience stigma and discrimination and are denied their human rights. By examining some of these complexities, the chapter aims to provide an introduction to sexual and reproductive

DOI: 10.4324/9781003408765-8

health and human rights and to trigger readers to think critically about key challenges, particularly those pertaining to the at times implicit and hidden root causes of human rights violations faced by "othered" individuals.

Learning Objectives

After studying this chapter you will be able to:

- Understand the (development of) key elements in sexual and reproductive health and rights
- Position sexual and reproductive health and rights within the international human rights framework
- Understand key gendered and compounding challenges to ensuring the highest standard of sexual and reproductive health
- Explore your own perspective and position on the right to safe abortion in the context of health and human rights

Changing Narratives on Sexual and Reproductive Health and Rights

Sexual and reproductive health (SRH) is an essential component of the WHO definition of health, which encompasses "a state of complete physical, mental and social well-being, and not merely the absence of disease or infirmity", as defined in the WHO Constitution (WHO, n.d.a). At the core of well-being lies health and bodily integrity. SRH, therefore, is crucially linked to the right to health. When people's health and bodily integrity are violated, it constitutes a violation of their human rights. The prevailing narratives surrounding SRH have evolved over time and vary depending on historical context and cultural perspectives. Understanding some of these key shifts is vital for comprehending the complex interplay among reproductive health, sexual health and human rights on the international stage.

Before the 1990s, issues related to sexual and reproductive health mainly focused on controlling women's fertility with the objective of controlling population growth. The narrative was thus defined following a population control paradigm, meaning that population control specialists and demographers played key roles in international consensus meetings dedicated to deliberating on reproductive health. This reflects that, at that time, reproduction was not understood and was addressed not as a matter of human rights but as a matter of demography (see Berro Pizzarossa, 2018). Various beliefs shaped this narrative; perhaps the most influential was the belief that poverty was mainly due to population growth and that the latter was thus the main barrier to development. As such, the need to control conception rates was understood as a priority to overcome this barrier.

Reproductive health was linked to human rights for the first time in a global agreement during the International Conference on Human Rights in 1968, 20 years after the adoption of the UDHR. The Tehran Proclamation affirmed the basic right of parents "to determine freely and responsibly the number and the spacing of their children" (Par. 16). However, population growth was still seen as a key barrier to the enjoyment of human rights, leaving space for population control mechanisms in the realisation of human rights (Berro Pizzarossa, 2018). Government responses adopted this narrative leading to expansion of family planning programmes and at times coercive interventions to reduce conception and lower fertility rates. Women were the primary target of population control programmes, following the assumption that, if the fertility of women is under control, population growth could be reduced. In 1984, two major controversies emerged during the second international conference on population in Mexico City. The first was US President Ronald Reagan's announcement of the "Mexico City Policy", which restricted international aid funding for family planning to organisations that excluded (information on) abortion from their services. The second was China's "one-child policy", which involved coercive population control methods by the Chinese government. These developments highlighted the disparity between the aforementioned international commitments and the actual political will of states to implement these rights and thus the lived realities among populations.

The population control narrative was turned on its head in 1994 giving rise to the narrative on sexual and reproductive health *and rights,* commonly referred to by the acronym SRHR. Representatives of 179 governments gathered in Cairo for the International Conference on Population and Development (ICPD) to draft a new consensus on responding to population growth. During this conference, it was agreed that population and development are inextricably linked. At ICPD it was asserted that the dignity, needs and rights of individuals were central in achieving fertility goals, rather than demographic targets and population control. This implied that, for the first time in a moment of international consensus, nations affirmed that reproductive health and rights stand as quintessential human rights, firmly established in both national and international legal frameworks.

This landmark conference placed reproductive rights on the global agenda – which was fundamental for global development – and recognised gender equality and women's empowerment to be central pillars to the sustainable development agenda. The ICPD made clear that SRHR are a crucial and essential element for the enjoyment of other human rights. The Programme of Action (PoA) adopted during this conference reaffirmed that reproductive rights *are not a new set of rights*, rather a collection of freedoms and entitlements that were already recognised in national laws, international human rights instruments and other consensus documents. The shift to recognise sexual and reproductive health as part of human rights can be attributed to the work of civil society organisations, non-governmental organisations, women's (rights) organisations and feminist scholars and activists who were active during the ICPD. Consequently, the empowerment of women and the promotion of rights in relation to reproduction were seen a key objective for family planning efforts at that time.

At ICPD it was acknowledged that empowering women and girls – and ensuring access to education and health care, including reproductive health – is crucial to safeguarding human rights. Central to this paradigm shift is the commitment to uphold and advance the human rights of women and girls. The PoA provided a definition of reproductive health, reproductive rights and reproductive health care (Chapter 7, 7.2), which are acknowledged and used to date.

Reproductive health:

> is a state of complete physical, mental and social well-being and not merely the absence of disease or infirmity, in all matters relating to the reproductive system

and to its functions and processes. Reproductive health therefore implies that people are able to have a satisfying and safe sex life and that they have the capability to reproduce and the freedom to decide if, when and how often to do so. Implicit in this last condition are the right of men and women to be informed and to have access to safe, effective, affordable and acceptable methods of family planning of their choice, as well as other methods of their choice for regulation of fertility which are not against the law, and the right of access to appropriate health-care services that will enable women to go safely through pregnancy and childbirth and provide couples with the best chance of having a healthy infant. In line with the above definition of reproductive health, reproductive health care is defined as the constellation of methods, techniques and services that contribute to reproductive health and well-being by preventing and solving reproductive health problems. It also includes sexual health, the purpose of which is the enhancement of life and personal relations, and not merely counselling and care related to reproduction and sexually transmitted diseases.

(ICPD PoA, Para. 7.2)

Reproductive rights:

embrace certain human rights that are already recognised in national laws, international human rights documents and other consensus documents. These rights rest on the recognition of the basic right of all couples and individuals to decide freely and responsibly the number, spacing and timing of their children, to have the information and means to do so, and the right to attain the highest standard of sexual and reproductive health. It also includes their right to make decisions concerning reproduction free of discrimination, coercion and violence, as expressed in human rights documents.

(ICPD PoA, Para. 7.3)

As is noticeable in these definitions, they are broad and encompass various interconnected elements. As we have progressed through time after ICPD, the elements established as part of SRHR have been – and continue to be – contested and debated. International consensus regarding subdomains has proven difficult and has proven particularly salient in the context of abortion, sexual health and rights including sexual orientation and identity. Such tensions were also present during the ICPD, leading to a compromise pertaining to abortion. The previous definition refers to one's access to family planning methods of choice, "which are not against the law", thereby excluding abortion services in countries outlawing these services (Starrs & Anderson, 2016). The Guttmacher-*Lancet* Commission argues that, as a consequence, initiatives in health and development have typically focused on particular components of SRHR such as: maternal mortality and health, newborn health, HIV/AIDS and contraception, whereas contributions to other areas such as gender-based violence (GBV), sexual and gender orientation and identity and access to safe medical abortion services have been limited (Starrs et al., 2018).

On the basis of various agreements, WHO reports – and the international human rights framework – the Guttmacher-*Lancet* Commission articulated an integrated definition of SRHR. In line with this definition, they articulated what essential SRHR interventions entail. The definition and related essential services read as follows:

> sexual and reproductive health is a state of physical, emotional, mental, and social wellbeing in relation to all aspects of sexuality and reproduction, not merely the absence of disease, dysfunction, or infirmity. Therefore, a positive approach to sexuality and reproduction should recognise the part played by pleasurable sexual relationships, trust, and communication in the promotion of self-esteem and overall wellbeing. All individuals have a right to make decisions governing their bodies and to access services that support that right. Achievement of sexual and reproductive health relies on the realisation of sexual and reproductive rights, which are based on the human rights of all individuals to: have their bodily integrity, privacy, and personal autonomy respected;
>
>> freely define their own sexuality, including sexual orientation and gender identity and expression;
>>
>> decide whether and when to be sexually active;
>>
>> choose their sexual partners;
>>
>> have safe and pleasurable sexual experiences;
>>
>> decide whether, when, and whom to marry;
>>
>> decide whether, when, and by what means to have a child or children, and how many children to have;
>>
>> have access over their lifetimes to the information, resources, services, and support necessary to achieve all the above, free from discrimination, coercion, exploitation, and violence.
>>
>> Essential sexual and reproductive health services must meet public health and human rights standards, including the "Availability, Accessibility, Acceptability, and Quality" framework of the right to health. The services should include:
>>
>> ■ accurate information and counselling on sexual and reproductive health, including evidence-based, comprehensive sexuality education;
>> ■ information, counselling, and care related to sexual function and satisfaction;
>> ■ prevention, detection, and management of sexual and gender-based violence and coercion;
>> ■ a choice of safe and effective contraceptive methods;
>> ■ safe and effective antenatal, childbirth, and postnatal care;
>> ■ safe and effective abortion services and care;
>> ■ prevention, management, and treatment of infertility;
>> ■ prevention, detection, and treatment of sexually transmitted infections, including HIV, and of reproductive tract infections; and
>> ■ prevention, detection, and treatment of reproductive cancers.
>
> *(Starrs et al., 2018)*

This definition of SRHR affirms that SRHR is not exclusive to women and includes men's health needs related to male reproductive organs such as sexually transmitted infections (STIs), infertility, erectile dysfunction or testicular or prostate cancers, as well as the rights of the LGBTQI+ community. Further, in their roles as partners, husbands, fathers and members of the household as well as leaders in the community, boys and men have duties as well as rights within SRHR.

SRHR in the Human Rights Framework

Within the international human rights framework, progress has been made to safeguard the human right to health following principles of autonomy, dignity, equality (non-discrimination) and security. The UDHR (UN, 1948) clearly states that human rights are universal, on the basis of one's humanity. Article 2 states; "Everyone is entitled to all the rights and freedoms set forth in this Declaration, without distinction of any kind, such as race, colour, sex, language, religion, political or other opinion, national or social origin, property, birth or other status". While the UDHR itself is not a legally binding treaty, it is the foundational document for the development of subsequent international human rights treaties and conventions. Key examples are the International Covenant on Civil and Political Rights (ICCPR) and the International Covenant on Economic, Social and Cultural Rights (ICESC), both of which were adopted in 1966. Together with the UDHR, these covenants are often referred to as the "International Bill of Human Rights". The principle of universality can be identified in the ICCPR and ICESC, as these affirm the equal rights of women and men and prohibit discrimination of any kind, including sex.

Chapter 1 addressed the development of the UDHR. However, it is important to add that the drafting of this document has been significantly influenced by a number of female delegates, who formed the UN Commission on the Status of Women (CSW). The CSW was established by council resolution 11(II) of June 21st in 1946 in order to promote, monitor and report on the status and rights of women. The CSW is the principal global intergovernmental body exclusively dedicated to the promotion of gender equality and the empowerment of women. Upon the conception of the CSW, all the representatives were women. As one of their first tasks, the commission ensured gender-sensitive and inclusive language in the UDHR. As noted in Chapter 1, the UDHR has often been criticised for being a "Western" framework. More recent work has told a different story and reflects on the drafting process, involving extensive debates among delegates from various backgrounds in order for the UDHR to, by design, accommodate for conflicting ideologies (Adami, 2018) (see Textbox 5.1).

Textbox 5.1
Contributors to the UDHR

The role of male and Western contributors to the UDHR has been well documented, as well as the contribution of Eleanor Roosevelt who was appointed as first Chairperson of the Commission on Human Rights and served a key role in drafting and completion of the UDHR. Importantly, other women also played critical roles in the shaping of this document which have been largely neglected. In the book *Women and the universal declaration of human rights*, Rebecca Adami questions the dominant Western, male narrative regarding the creation of human rights and, more specifically, the UDHR. Presenting a counter narrative, Adami highlights previously neglected role of the non-Western women, including female delegates from the Dominican Republic, India and Pakistan, who have had an influence on the drafting process. Delegates from different nations and cultural and religious backgrounds, as well as different beliefs on socials justice, extensively debated the UDHR in over 200 sessions. Consequently, they did not agree on a single correct or "right" basis for human rights but achieved consensus on a set of rights accommodating conflicting ideologies (Adami, 2018).

While a singular human rights document or treaty exclusively dedicated to SRHR does not exist, various international instruments, both within the UN and within regional and national contexts, protect elements of sexual and reproductive rights. These protections fall under the broader umbrella of ensuring "the highest attainable standard of health". However, SRHR are not fully encapsulated by – or limited to – the right to health as articulated in Article 25 of the UDHR, given that the human rights underlying SRHR are interrelated and interdependent. For instance, the "right to life", enshrined in Article 3 of the UDHR, which asserts "everyone has the right to life, liberty, and security of person", extends to include the prevention of maternal deaths. This implies that individuals require access to emergency obstetric health care as well as safe abortion services, among other maternal health services. The right to education (Article 26) necessitates access to age-appropriate information about sexuality for all individuals, regardless of age. Moreover, the commitment to non-discrimination (Article 2) prohibits the denial or criminalisation of sex-specific health services, constituting violations of human rights. Additionally, the right to health mandates that health services, including contraceptives, adhere to the principles of availability, accessibility, affordability, acceptability and good quality (AAAQ yardstick), as discussed in Chapter 3.

The following section will introduce some of the relevant human right standards – in addition to the ICPD introduced earlier in this chapter – that collectively contribute to the promotion and protection of sexual and reproductive health and rights worldwide. Note that this is not an exhaustive list of relevant standards.

The **1966** International Covenant on Civil and Political Rights (ICCPR) Article 6 and the International Covenant on Economic, Social and Cultural Rights (ICESCR) Article 12 affirm the right to life and the right to the highest attainable standard of physical and mental health, respectively.

In **1979**, the Convention on the Elimination of All Forms of Discrimination against Women (CEDAW) was adopted by the General Assembly, known as the 'Women's Bill of Rights' and came into force in 1981. CEDAW defines what constitutes discrimination against women and refers to

any distinction, exclusion or restriction made on the basis of sex which has the effect or purpose of impairing or nullifying the recognition, enjoyment or exercise by women, irrespective of their marital status, on a basis of equality of men and women, of human rights and fundamental freedoms in the political, economic, social, cultural, civil or any other field.

(Article 1)

This definition is broad in terms of scope ("any other field") and refers to indirect discrimination ("which has the effect"). The convention establishes an agenda for action to i) eradicate discriminatory laws, policies and practices; ii) to take affirmative measures and iii) to eradicate substantive discrimination. CEDAW emphasises equal access to healthcare services – and explicitly mentions family planning – in Article 12. It further ensures women's right to education, including specific information related to family planning (Article 10) and the freedom to decide on the number and spacing of their children and to have access to information and education (Article 16). CEDAW emphasises that women's health and reproductive rights are fundamental to achieving gender equality. This extends the principles of the Declaration of Alma-Ata (1978) which recognised maternal health, family planning and midwifery under primary health care policy. CEDAW has been signed by 189 states parties to date, with the exception of the United States, Sudan, Iran and Somalia. As compared to other treaties, CEDAW has received the largest number of reservations. A reservation allows a state to specify a part of the Convention that it does not agree to be bound by. Many countries have made reservations to various provisions of CEDAW, often due to conflicts with national laws, religious beliefs, or cultural practices. Bangladesh, Bahrain, Egypt, Iraq, Libya, Morocco, Syria and the United Arab Emirates made reservations to parts of the Convention, citing conflicts with Shari'a law. However, not all states that apply Shari'a law entered reservations while referring to Shari'a as the reason, meaning that interpretations vary and are inconsistent. These reservations often concerned (parts of) Article 2, Article 9 and Article 16, which concern condemning discrimination against women in all its forms (Article 2), equal rights for women in retaining and transferring their nationality to children (Article 9) and the equality of men and women in marriage and family relations (Article 16). These articles received most reservations, also by other countries, including Lesotho, New Zealand, Niger, Singapore and the UK, while they are argued by the CEDAW Committee to relate to fundamental aspects of the Convention to ensure non-discrimination.

The Convention on the Rights of the Child, effective since **1990**, ensures children's right to the highest attainable standard of health in Article 24 and ensures pre- and post-natal care for mothers as well as referencing family planning education and guidance for parents. Article 28 states the right of children to education.

Influenced by the women's rights lobby, the Vienna Declaration and Programme for Action (**1993**) emphasised the universality of all human rights and thereby highlighted that the rights of women are integral to the human rights framework. For instance, in Article 18 it states that "the human rights of women and of the girl-child are an inalienable, integral and indivisible part of universal human rights". The article further calls for the elimination of sex-based discrimination, GBV and all forms of sexual harassment and exploitation (UN, n.d.).

The Beijing Platform for Action established in **1995** during the Fourth World Conference on Women built upon and reaffirmed the language of the Vienna Declaration and the ICPD Platform for Action, as discussed at the beginning of this chapter. The Beijing Platform for Action is a progressive document for advancing women's rights and also refers to women's sexuality. It grants that "the human rights of women include their right to have control over and decide freely and responsibly on matters related to their sexuality, including sexual and reproductive health, free of coercion, discrimination and violence" (paragraph 96, PoA) (UN Women, 1995).

Additional important human rights obligations include the UN Committee on Economic, Social and Cultural Rights General Comment No. 22 on the right to sexual and reproductive health and the Sustainable Development Goals (SDGs). Goals 3, 4 and 5 are of particular relevance to SRHR. Goal 3 aims to ensure healthy lives and to promote well-being for all at all ages, directly encompassing sexual and reproductive health. It includes targets such as reducing maternal mortality and preventable deaths under five years of age, ending the AIDS epidemic and ensuring universal access to sexual and reproductive health services. Goal 4 ensures inclusive and equitable quality education and promotes lifelong learning opportunities for all. Comprehensive sexuality education is crucial for equipping individuals with knowledge about their SRHR, including contraception and healthy relationships. Goal 5 aims to achieve gender equality and empower all women and girls. Gender equality is fundamental to SRHR, a notion we will unpack further in this chapter. Goal 5 includes targets such as ending all forms of discrimination, eliminating all forms of violence against women and girls and eliminating harmful practices.

Last, Article 25 of the Convention on the Rights of Persons with Disabilities (CRPD), which was adopted in 2006, addresses the right to sexual and reproductive health for disabled persons.

Based on international human rights treaties and conventions, regional normative frameworks can be drafted to ensure human rights, including sexual and reproductive rights. For example, the European Union has drafted the "EU Charter of Fundamental Rights". While this charter does not explicitly include provisions in relation to sexual and reproductive health, it includes provisions in relation to dignity, the right to life and integrity of person (see Chapter 1). Further, Article 21 references non-discrimination, stating:

> any discrimination based on any ground such as sex, race, colour, ethnic or social origin, genetic features, language, religion or belief, political or any other opinion, membership of a national minority, property, birth, disability, age or sexual orientation shall be prohibited.

In 2014, the "Council of Europe Convention on preventing and combating violence against women and domestic violence", also known as the "Istanbul Convention", came into force, upon ten ratifications among which eight members were states of the Council of Europe. This convention is based on the notion that violence against women is a type of gender-based violence committed against women.

In 2013, Latin America and the Caribbean adopted the Montevideo consensus on population and development, a significant regional agreement, which reaffirmed the principles articulated in the ICPD PoA and highlighted universal access to sexual and reproductive health services as well as gender equality as part of their ten priority areas. The document states it is agreed to "Promote, protect and guarantee sexual health and rights and reproductive rights in order to contribute to the fulfilment of persons and to social justice in a society free from all forms of discrimination and violence" (Article

33). Further, it explicitly references sexual rights in Article 34, claiming to "promote policies that enable persons to exercise their sexual rights, which embrace the right to a safe and full sex life".

Another important example of a progressive regional document including sexual and reproductive rights is the "Protocol to the African Charter on Human and Peoples' Rights on the Rights of Women in Africa", also referred to as the "Maputo Protocol" and its related "Plan of Action of the African Union" (AU) (see Textbox 5.2). The protocol is distinguished by its forward-thinking approach, specifically via its prohibition of female genital mutilation, marriage of girls under 18 and forced marriage. It addresses all forms of public and private GBV and ensures legal protection of girls from sexual harassment and abuse. It affirms the right to health for girls and women, including SRH. Notably, it stands as the first protocol to recognise safe abortion under specific conditions as a human right and explicitly mentions HIV and AIDS. Last, the protocol is recognised for its acknowledgement of vulnerable and marginalised populations, such as adolescents, elderly women, widows, disabled women, women in poverty and migrant or refugee women (Van Eerdewijk et al., 2018).

Textbox 5.2
The Maputo Protocol

The protocol was adopted in 2003 and enforced in 2005. It stands as a landmark document for women's and girls' human rights across the African continent and globally. It addresses the gaps in the African Charter (1981) regarding women's and girls' rights, offering 32 articles dedicated to their rights. The protocol notably defines discrimination against women, a concept previously absent in the African Charter, as any differentiation, exclusion or restriction based on sex that undermines women's recognition, enjoyment or exercise of human rights and fundamental freedoms in all aspects of life, regardless of marital status. Women's rights organisations have been instrumental in the adoption of the Maputo Protocol and continue to advocate for its further ratification, adaptation and enforcement (Van Eerdewijk et al., 2018).

Progress and Common Violations of SRHR

Since the ICPD in 1994, significant strides have been made in enhancing and ensuring access to essential sexual and reproductive health services. This progress is evident through various indicators across SRHR health domains. For example, the WHO reports that Eastern Europe and Southern Asia achieved a decline of 70% (38 to 11) and 67% (408 to 134) in maternal mortality ratio (MMR) between 2000 and 2020. The MMR refers to the number of maternal deaths per number of live births. Countries in Sub-Saharan Africa also, on average, reduced their MMR by 33% in this timeframe (WHO, 2024a). Further, the global adolescent birth rate (ABR) has decreased from 64.5 births per 1,000 women (from 15–19 years) in 2000 to 41.3 births per 1,000 women in 2023 (WHO, 2024b). The number of users of modern contraceptives has nearly doubled since 1990. While progress is undeniable, health inequities in this health domain persist:

- Every day in 2020, almost 800 women died from preventable causes related to pregnancy and childbirth, and 95% of maternal deaths happen in lower- and middle-income countries (WHO, 2024a). Further, pregnancy or childbirth complications are among the leading causes of deaths for girls aged 15–19 years old, globally (WHO, 2023a).
- Globally, one in three women on average have been subjected to either physical and/or sexual intimate partner violence or non-partner sexual violence. Most of this violence is perpetrated by intimate partners (WHO, 2024c).
- In 2022, 39 million people were living with HIV and 480,000 young people (between 10–24 years old) were newly infected with HIV, of whom 140,000 were adolescents (10–19 years old). Globally, 75% of new HIV infections among adolescents occur among girls (UNICEF, 2023).
- Worldwide, only one in two adolescent girls and young women (between 15–19 years old) have their family planning demands met by modern methods (UNICEF, 2023)
- Reproductive health and rights continue to be a topic of debate. A total of 24 countries in the world completely prohibit abortion, while over 50 countries only permit abortions in case of risk to the woman's health. Globally, 25 million unsafe abortions are occurring each year (Starrs et al., 2018). Moreover, 45% of all abortions are unsafe (WHO, 2024d).
- Forced, coercive or involuntary sterilisation, involving the sterilisation without informed consent, has a long history and continues to target individuals with a disability, mental illness, racialised or Indigenous individuals, women with HIV, women in poverty and transgender and intersex persons (WHO, 2014).

In addition to some of the health inequities presented earlier that are particularly salient among certain groups of people (e.g., girls, women, gender-diverse populations, adolescents, disabled people, racialised populations), the progress in SRHR has been uneven between world regions. Maternal mortality remains unacceptably high in some areas of the world, with lower-income countries reporting an average MMR of 430/100,000 live births while this is 13/100,000 in higher income countries (WHO, 2024a). In South Sudan, Chad and Nigeria, MMR is rated as extremely high with over 1,000 maternal deaths per 100,000 live births (WHO et al., 2023). These deaths occur due to complications during or following pregnancy and childbirth. In most cases these are preventable. Some of the major complications include severe bleeding, infections, high blood pressure during pregnancy, delivery complications and unsafe abortions (WHO, 2024a). Moreover, pregnancies among adolescents appear to be more frequent among individuals with a low economic status or less education. Further, ABRs are highest in Sub-Saharan African, Latin American and Caribbean countries (WHO, 2024b). While abortion care is included in the essential health care services list by the WHO, abortion remains a highly debated, contested and stigmatised health services domain, leading to a lack of access to timely, safe, affordable and quality abortion services (WHO, 2024d). It is thus safe to conclude that, currently, the SRHR agenda remains unfinished.

Changes in political leadership, as well as international humanitarian crises such as natural disasters, conflicts or pandemics can reveal the fragility of our sexual and reproductive health systems and services. What we have learned from previous crises is that, when things go wrong in the world, progress within SRH can be swiftly reversed. These crises have laid bare the far-reaching consequences this can have on the SRH of individuals, families and communities, with girls, women and gender-diverse populations often being disproportionately impacted. A key example of changes in political leadership and impact on SRHR is the reinstatement of the controversial "Mexico City Policy" or so-called "Global Gag Rule" by the Trump administration, shortly after President Trump took office in 2017. This policy prohibited the allocation of federal US funding to non-governmental organisations and agencies that provide, promote or refer to abortion services or even provide information about abortions. Studies have reported, as a result of the reinstatement of this policy, funding cuts; increased abortion rates, maternal mortality and morbidity and reduced access to STI, contraception and peri-natal services across various contexts (see for example Lane et al., 2021).

Further, a global pandemic or humanitarian crises like war or natural disasters can disrupt the essential health care infrastructure, including facilities, supply chains and personnel, making it challenging for individuals to access critical health services, including SRH services. The displacement of populations and breakdown of social systems can increase exposure to different forms of violence and exacerbate existing inequities. During the outbreak of COVID-19, for example, health systems became overwhelmed with the demand to care for COVID-19 patients, and previously accessible SRH services were suddenly suspended. In addition, fear, misconceptions and activity restrictions surrounding the pandemic hampered access to care. A systematic review found that the majority of LMICs did not manage to ensure SRHR in the response to COVID-19 due to increasing restrictions and limited resources (Singh et al., 2023). It is important that SRHR are incorporated in emergency preparedness and humanitarian response planning in all countries, in order to safeguard access to essential services and mitigate indirect impacts (Maier et al., 2021; Singh et al., 2023), as well as ensuring the provision of a comprehensive set of services designated as essential SRH services.

Gender and Sexual and Reproductive Health
SRH is linked to equitable gender relations and thus the principle of non-discrimination. Before diving into the process and outcomes of gendered SRH inequities, it is useful to clearly distinguish between definitions of sex and gender. According to the WHO, sex is defined as "the biological characteristics that define humans as female or male. While these sets of biological characteristics are not mutually exclusive, as there are individuals who possess both, they tend to differentiate humans as males and females" (WHO, n.d.b). Gender is defined as "the characteristics of women, men, girls and boys that are socially constructed. This includes norms, behaviours and roles associated with being a woman, man, girl or boy, as well as relationships with each other" (WHO, n.d.b). Further, gender norms have been defined as the "unspoken rules that govern the attributes and behaviours that are valued and considered acceptable for men, women and gender minorities" (Heise et al., 2019, p. 2441).

SRHR are influenced by both biological sex and gender, affecting health risks, access to and outcomes of SRH services. However, there is an important distinction to be made between when health outcomes are *different* or when they are *inequitable* and, in the latter case, thus become an issue of human rights. For example, persons that are determined to be biologically female at birth can experience menstruation and pregnancy and may be at risk for health conditions like endometriosis or cervical cancer or for contracting certain STIs, such as HIV. Health outcomes that are rooted in biological sex thereby refer to health differences. Gender systems[1] may influence the consequences of such health differences and, in turn, health inequities are produced by gender inequality and other axes of oppression (Braveman & Gruskin, 2003). Specifically, gender systems contribute to the creation of health inequities through the social production of gender, determining an individual's social position, which lead to gendered pathways to health including gendered differences in exposure, health behaviours, impacts in accessing care, biased health systems and biased health research, institutions and data collection which can create health inequities (Heise et al., 2019).

Simone de Beauvoir on Gender: "One Is Not Born, But Rather Becomes, a Woman"

Before looking further into the creation of gendered health inequities within SRH, the chapter first introduces the work of Simone de Beauvoir to help understand the concept of gender and gender inequality. Simone de Beauvoir's seminal work *The Second Sex* was published in 1949. De Beauvoir was a French existentialist[2] thinker and her work has had a vast influence on feminist thought and continues to shape our perceptions of gender, as well as our self- and relational conceptions, to this day. De Beauvoir departs from the notion that all individuals are fundamentally free and thus not defined by social, economic, geographical or political conditions. She argues that, since individuals are ontologically free, people are not defined by their sex. A key point from her work is thus the distinction of gender from essentialist boundaries of biological sex. De Beauvoir posits that gender is a social construct you are "made into" through a process of "becoming" by acculturation. She highlighted that being a woman is not a biological fact which is genetically determined at birth but extends beyond this as a process of identity formation and socialisation within a specific social and cultural context. She thereby critiques the essentialist perspective that women are defined by their reproductive capability and argues that womanhood is shaped by cultural and social factors over time. Gender is thereby understood as socially constructed and as an identity that individuals can actively negotiate within the framework of social norms and expectations.

De Beauvoir further critiques and reflects on the impact of Aristotle's view on humanity. Aristotle was convinced that women should be seen as "unfinished or defective men", with biological and rational capacities inferior to those of men, limited to their capacity to reproduce. This explicit notion of male supremacy established men and masculinity as the norm, casting women and femininity into the realm of the "other". De Beauvoir argues that women are thus defined *in relation to* men, rather than as autonomous and rational beings, in which the female gender is considered inferior to the male gender. To illustrate this, she stated; "man is defined as a human being and women as a female, whenever she behaves as a human being she is said to imitate the male". She thereby references the implicit yet default normative construction of humanity as "male" or "masculine". In turn, female inferiority poses challenges for achieving humanity – and by extension universal human rights – for anyone who does not fit hegemonic masculine norms.

This chapter argues that this process of othering continues to lead to bias and limitations in our understanding of health and care in contemporary societies, particularly for girls, women and gender diverse individuals. This requires urgent attention given that it limits these groups' ability to achieve the highest attainable standard of health (Heise et al., 2019; Jaffee et al., 2016). While there are several gendered pathways to health which create health inequity, as also discussed by Heise and colleagues, this chapter specifically reflects on some of the biases present in health research and health systems, including patient–provider interactions.

Bias in Research

The implicit normative construction of humanity as male continues to impact medical and health research. The systematic underfunding and lack of attention to research into women's sex-specific health issues as well as the limited integration of sex and gender considerations in general health research have resulted in a lack of, incomplete or biased understanding of (sexual and reproductive) health and treatments (WHO, 2009). For instance, there are persistent gaps in knowledge regarding certain sex-specific health conditions which may hamper diagnosis and access to care. See, for example, the case of endometriosis in Textbox 5.3. Furthermore, many health conditions or treatments are assumed to be gender neutral, meaning that these are assumed to affect different individuals in the same way, regardless of sex or gender. Historically, women have been largely excluded from clinical trials which was largely attributed to woman's hormone cycle and justified to protect (pregnant) women from risks related to research. Hormone cycles would supposedly make women imperfect candidates for studies. In the US, it was not until 1993 that researchers were legally obliged to include women in their research (McGovern, 1997).

While research on women's health as well as promotion of balanced sex/gender representation and analysis has been improving and increasing, challenges persist. Sex- and gender-based analysis can be challenged by conceptual, methodological and data challenges, and reporting of results by sex remains limited (Parekh et al., 2011; Runnels et al., 2014). We are thus confronted with gaps in our understanding regarding how health conditions or certain treatments affect individuals differently. For instance, male bias has been reported to persist in drug development and biomedical research (Beery & Zucker, 2011). A systematic review of a random sample of clinical randomised controlled trials (RCTs) from high-impact journals found an overrepresentation of men in 43% of the studies, and only 39% of the RCTs included an equal division between men and women (Phillips & Hamber, 2016). Moreover, studies have indicated that women tend to be at higher risk of adverse drug reactions (de Vries et al., 2019; Parekh et al., 2011), and that women are differently or disproportionately affected by certain conditions such as cardiovascular disease or autoimmune diseases. As such, this holds relevance beyond SRH. Since these are important issues in women's health but beyond the scope of this chapter, additional references to studies on some of such health disparities are included at the end of this chapter for further reading.

Textbox 5.3 presents a short case study on endometriosis and the implications of the lack of knowledge on treatment and health outcomes of individuals who are affected by this health condition.

Textbox 5.3
Case Study: Endometriosis

Endometriosis is a chronic gynaecological health condition which presents through chronic pelvic pain, painful menstruation and heavy bleeding, painful sex and infertility. While research on endometriosis is now increasing, the condition has been largely ignored in research funding, leading to gaps in understanding of its aetiology, associated symptoms and impact on one's daily life. This has detrimental impacts on the lives of individuals who are affected by endometriosis.

In the US, a diagnosis can take more than 7 years, which is found to be even longer for Black women (Bougie et al., 2019). Furthermore, there is limited research on the social factors that impact the well-being of those affected by endometriosis (Kocas et al., 2023). Studies have shown that endometriosis is associated with stigma, with women facing disbelief and ignorance from health professionals, leading to delays in diagnosis and a lack of appropriate care (Matías-González et al., 2021; Seear, 2009). Women's symptoms are frequently discredited and normalised as part of menstrual pain, which plays a significant role in the trivialisation and normalisation of their pain (Seear, 2009). Another study among Puerto Rican women with endometriosis revealed similar findings, indicating that women were stigmatised and blamed for excessive whining or complaining (Matías-González et al., 2021).

Questions for Discussion

Individually or in a group, discuss

- What specific challenges might different individuals face that contribute to diagnostic delays?
- Different ways you can identify how the process of "othering" has contributed to the health outcomes highlighted in the case study.

Bias in Health Systems: Gender Stereotyping and Decision-making

Throughout *The Second Sex*, de Beauvoir critiques the myths and beliefs surrounding the female gender and femininity and argues that such myths undermine women's freedom. In social psychology, such knowledge structures or beliefs have been conceptualised as "stereotypes". The field of social psychology has extensively studied stereotyping, identifying stereotypes as knowledge structures or beliefs regarding the characteristics of an individual or those of a group (Dovidio et al., 2010; Hilton & Von Hippel, 1996; Stangor, 2009). In and of themselves, stereotypes are not necessarily negative or harmful, since they can help us make sense of the world. Stereotypes can relate to certain characteristics such as physical or behavioural traits, clothing and social roles. They can serve a useful purpose as they can help us understand others or groups who are unfamiliar to us. For instance, at a public event or at the scene of an accident, a medic's uniform ensures they stand out to both bystanders and authorities, facilitating swift access and response. Stereotypes can exist without people agreeing with them and they can be positive, neutral or negative. However, when an individual endorses a negative stereotype, this turns into prejudice. Prejudice comprises a negative emotional response or attitude towards a person or a group and can ultimately result in discriminatory behaviours and actions. Important to note is that even neutral stereotypes may be harmful in situations where they strip decision-making power from the person being stereotyped.

Gender stereotypes are deeply ingrained in our society, shaping our understanding and expectations of the roles we should occupy within society, communities, families and relationships, as well as the principles governing how people should behave. Such stereotypes do not suddenly disappear during our interactions with the health system and thus can also shape access to – and decision-making in – health care (Travis et al., 2012). To illustrate this, a US-based study found that feminine stereotypes were typically characterised by kindness, sensitivity and patience (Prentice & Carranza, 2002). These tend to align better with a focus on health, both one's own and that of others, which relates to health-seeking behaviours (Lyons, 2009; Pattyn et al., 2015). In contrast, masculine stereotypes generally emphasised qualities such as assertiveness, competitiveness, ambition and self-reliance, which tend to be associated with lower health-seeking behaviours (Courtenay, 2000; Pattyn et al., 2015). Such prescriptive gender stereotypes are not static; they evolve over time and vary across different contexts.

The practice of gender stereotyping has been acknowledged as a human rights violation (see the work by Cook & Cusack, 2010; Cusack, 2013) and has been identified as an issue for urgent attention in a 2013 report submitted to the Office of the High Commissioner for Human Rights (OHCHR), titled "Gender Stereotyping as a Human Rights Violation". Cook and Cusack state that a stereotype becomes problematic and, in fact, a human rights issue when a stereotype "operates to ignore individuals' characteristics, abilities, needs, wishes, and circumstances in ways that deny individuals their human rights and fundamental freedoms, and when it creates gender hierarchies" (Cook & Cusack, 2010, p. 20). They distinguish between gender *stereotyping* – referring to a practice – and gender *stereotypes*, described as an umbrella term for a set of views or beliefs. Gender stereotypes include sex-role stereotypes (e.g., women take care of the family and men are breadwinners), sex stereotypes (e.g., women are weak, men are aggressive), sexual stereotypes (e.g., women are sexually passive, men have higher libidos) and compounded stereotypes (e.g., women with disabilities are asexual). See Textbox 5.4 for the relevant full definitions.

Textbox 5.4
Gender Stereotyping Definitions

- **Gender stereotyping** refers to the "practice of ascribing to an individual woman or man specific attributes, characteristics, or roles by reason only of her or his membership in the social group of women or men" (Cusack, 2013, p. 9).
- A **gender stereotype** has been defined as "a generalised view or preconception about attributes or characteristics that are or ought to be possessed by, or the roles that are or should be performed by, men and women" (Cusack, 2013, p. 8).
- A **compounded stereotype** is defined as "a generalised view or preconception about groups that result from the ascription of attributes, characteristics or roles based on one or more other traits, for example sex/gender and disability" (Cusack, 2013, p. 15).

In reality, it is difficult to generalise men, women and gender diverse people such as non-binary persons or transgender individuals each into their own group. The social position of a human being is always determined by multiple social determinants such as one's age, socioeconomic status or ethnicity, as well as one's geographic location, which may grant privilege or oppression depending on the context of the individual. Many of the stereotypes labelled as gender stereotypes are thus *compounded gender stereotypes*, as they pertain to specific individuals or groups of women, such as adolescent women, women of childbearing age, black women or women with disabilities, rather than women as a whole (Cook & Cusack, 2010; Cusack, 2013). Compounded gender stereotypes thus exert their core effects on the well-being of individuals through *compounded discrimination*, commonly referred to as "intersectional discrimination". For instance, gender discrimination intersects with discrimination due to one's health status, needs or disability, as well as with other parts of one's identity, like ethnicity or class. Intersecting forms of discrimination are increasingly addressed in global health, rooted in black feminist thought and scholarship (see Textbox 5.5).

Textbox 5.5
Intersectionality

Intersectional thinking can be traced back to over 50 years ago, and terms used over time have been "double jeopardy" by Frances Beal (1969), "interlocking systems of oppression" by the Combahee River Collective (1977) or the "matrix of domination" by Patricia Hill Collins (1990). Furthermore, Audre Lorde – a poet, essayist and feminist of African American descent – also addressed the interconnected forms of oppression in her activism and in her writings. The term "intersectionality" was coined by Kimberlé Crenshaw in 1989. She aimed to shed light on the intersection between race and gender, recognising the unique disadvantage and oppression faced by black women in the legal system in the US (Crenshaw, 1989). Intersectional thinking challenged prior "single-issue" social movements, such as the gender-only focus of the feminist movement at the time. Intersectional thinking historically focused on interlocking systems and structures of power that influence one's social position, shaped by multiple interconnected social identities, such as gender, class or ethnicity. A critical takeaway is that forms of oppression have compounded impacts on individuals, groups and communities and thus do not exist separately from each other. Therefore, if we aim to better understand human experiences, these should not be reduced to a single social category, given that social categories interact and mutually construct one another (Crenshaw, 1989; Collins & Bilge, 2016; Hankivsky, 2012).

The urgency to take into account and address gender stereotyping in health was acknowledged by the CEDAW committee, which stated that gender stereotyping may negatively affect women's decision-making regarding their health care, their sexuality and their reproductive health, impacting autonomy. The committee argued that States Parties to the UN should address harmful stereotypes and eliminate wrongful gender stereotyping. Two international human rights treaties include obligations that address harmful stereotypes and wrongful stereotyping including Article 5 of CEDAW and Article 8(1)(b) of the CRPD.

Article 5 states:

> parties shall take all appropriate measures . . . to modify the social and cultural patterns of conduct of men and women, with a view to achieving the elimination of prejudices and customary and all other practices which are based on the idea of the inferiority or the superiority of either of the sexes or on stereotyped roles for men and women.

Article 8(1)(b) states:

> parties undertake to adopt immediate, effective and appropriate measures to combat stereotypes, prejudices and harmful practices relating to persons with disabilities, including those based on sex and age, in all areas of life.

Common Gender Stereotypes and Impact on SRH

Despite the significant and continued detrimental impact of gender stereotyping and discrimination, the practice is often misunderstood, overlooked or disregarded in health care (Travis et al., 2012). Moreover, given that some pervasive stereotypes and gender relations are considered "normal", this obscures how such beliefs, attitudes, behaviours and structural factors determine who benefits from health systems and interactions and frameworks of research. This leads to structurally overlooking groups that are othered.

Specifically, stereotypes can lead to disregarding girls' and women's abilities, characteristics, needs and desires, thereby stripping them of their agency, autonomy and decision-making power, perpetuating barriers to equitable health outcomes and reproductive rights and reinforcing gender hierarchies (O'Connell & Zampas, 2018). To exemplify the impact of compounded stereotypes, three common stereotypes – as also raised by Cook and Cusack (2010) – and their potential impacts on SRHR are discussed here, including;

1. Women as mothers and/or caretakers
2. Women as irrational, vulnerable and/or weak
3. Women as sexually modest/chaste/submissive

First, the stereotype of women as caregivers and/or mothers is common across contexts across the globe. While this stereotype is not inherently hostile, it can have negative consequences by diminishing women's and mothers' autonomy in decision-making and overshadowing other aspects of their identity. This, for instance, can restrict their opportunities beyond domestic roles and result in women expected to assume all caregiving responsibilities within a family (Cook & Cusack, 2010). Frances Raday, a former member of the UN Committee on the Elimination of Discrimination Against Women (CEDAW), highlighted this issue in 2007:

> the most globally pervasive of the harmful cultural practices . . . is the stereotyping of women exclusively as mothers and housewives in a way that limits their opportunities to participate in public life, whether political or economic. . . .

Stereotypical assignment of sole or major responsibility for childcare to women disadvantages women across cultures.

(Raday, 2007)

Moreover, this stereotype can facilitate beliefs that women are destined to become mothers, reinforcing the notion that they should carry any pregnancy to term regardless of circumstances. This belief not only emphasises the importance of protecting foetal health under any circumstance – endangering the life of the pregnant person – but it can also restrict access to contraception in the context of marriage. Further, this stereotype can fuel the stigmatisation of women who are childless or face challenges in conceiving (Whiteford & Gonzalez, 1995).

Second, the stereotype that women are irrational, vulnerable and/or weak is associated with the assumption that women are incapable of making rational decisions or accurately report their symptoms. This can inform paternalistic policies that restrict reproductive choices and undermine women's autonomy and informed consent in health (Cook & Cusack, 2010). For example, Manian (2009) describes how such beliefs can justify state intervention to deny abortion services, undermining women's autonomy. Manian further highlighted how seeing women as weak can lead to the denial of services through a "women-protective rationale". Following this rationale, women are in need of protection, which may lead to a denial of services. Take, for example, the denial of abortion services, which can be justified as protecting women by preventing regret and depression (Cook & Cusack, 2010). An introduction and discussion of the lack of access to safe abortion services and the work of a women's organisation in providing access is provided by the case study in Textbox 5.6. Additionally, the "women are irrational" stereotype can contribute to the dismissal of women's health concerns. Consequently, women's descriptions of pain or symptoms may be deemed exaggerated or not credible. A 2021 study found that the assumption that women complain more can have consequences for their health, as their ability to accurately report pain can be underestimated (Zhang et al., 2021). Another 2020 study found that male doctors are more likely to underestimate pain when their patient is female (Miron-Shatz et al., 2020). Such stereotypes can be compounded by other social positions. For example, people of colour have been found to be significantly more likely to be undertreated for pain, regardless of their pain (Green et al., 2003).

Third, the stereotype of women as sexually modest, chaste and/or submissive can erode their agency and autonomy in sexual encounters and hinder access to SRH care. Such stereotypes fuel stigmatisation of certain health conditions. For instance, an HIV infection is often associated with promiscuity. In many cultures, this does not align with appropriate behaviour for women, driving stigma. Poor health outcomes can thus be exacerbated, as the fear of HIV-related stigma may deter women from disclosure or seeking health services in order to preserve their "womanhood" (Ojikutu et al., 2016; Yang et al., 2021).

Furthermore, the expectation of sexual submission can reinforce harmful attitudes that objectify individuals and contribute to instances of sexual violence and rape. In the context of marital rape, this stereotype may foster the belief that a woman's consent within marriage is implicit or irrelevant, leading to the dismissal of her autonomy and bodily integrity. Marital rape is a grave form of domestic violence and a violation of human rights. However, this stereotype is so pervasive that, in some countries, marital rape is not criminalised (Van Eerdewijk et al., 2018). Additionally, survivors of GBV may face discrimination due to prevailing assumptions that woman experiencing violence would have violated gendered and marital expectations (Barnett et al., 2016).

These compounded stereotypes highlighted here thus lie at the root of multidimensional othering and stigmatisation of individuals and their health and well-being, leading to bias in health research and health care, perpetuating poor health outcomes. This process undermines girls' and women's human rights. It is crucial that researchers, universities, government bodies, (women's) human rights institutions and non-governmental organisations gather insights on the various realities and nuanced differences in needs of men, women and gender diverse individuals to challenge bias and stereotyping in health systems and research. We have to recognise that, even when laws and policies are in place to combat stereotypes, these stereotypes can still impact health research and health care, for instance, through the type of research questions raised by researchers, the research proposals that receive funding or the interactions between health care professionals and patients. These impacts are often not immediately apparent or consciously recognised.

Textbox 5.6
Case Study: Access to Abortion Services

Globally, an estimated 56 million induced abortions occur annually, with approximately 25% of pregnancies ending in abortion. Abortion remains one of the most contentious and highly regulated medical procedures. Despite its prevalence, access to safe abortion services varies widely, leading to significant disparities in reproductive health care and rights. While some countries have legalised abortion, many still enforce strict laws, creating social inequality and endangering women's health.

Access to safe abortion services is particularly challenging for those without financial resources, driving them to seek unsafe alternatives. The medicines used for a medical abortion, mifepristone and misoprostol, have been on the list of essential medicines of the WHO since 2005 and are available in almost all European countries, the USA, Russia, China, Australia and Canada (WHO, 2023b). Even though abortion pills have been available for more than 25 years and are as safe as commonly used painkillers available over the counter (National Academies of Sciences, 2018), most countries do not allow telemedical abortion services and self-use of abortion pills.

Founded in 1999, a Dutch non-profit organisation called Women on Waves has been a pioneer in challenging restrictive laws and providing innovative solutions to ensure access to safe abortion. They collaborate closely with Women on Web, utilising subversive legal strategies to challenge restrictive abortion laws. Their initiatives include abortion ships, safe abortion hotlines, a safe abortion app, abortion drone deliveries and strategic litigation. Women on Waves has catalysed policy changes and increased awareness about safe abortion options globally. Their efforts have had far-reaching effects on reproductive health care and policy reform. Scientific studies have demonstrated the safety and acceptability of telemedical abortion services, leading to increased recognition and adoption of similar initiatives worldwide. Notably, Women on Waves' expertise in finding legal loopholes and use subversive legal strategies are intended to influence policies. For example, the ships campaign resulted in the legalisation of abortion in Portugal; the safe abortion hotlines are now run by organisations trained by Women on Waves, usually youth-led, and they have become important actors on the public debate in their countries, advocating and leading towards fundamental change at the grassroots level. The first hotlines set up by Women on Waves now initiate and train new hotlines in other countries.

Questions for Discussion

■ Argue your position and engage with counterarguments in relation to the following statement: "all people who can get pregnant should have access to medical abortion services".

■ Argue your position in regard to the following case: In a country, the government has passed a law restricting access to abortion, making it available only in cases where the life of the pregnant person is at risk. Human rights organisations and advocates assert that restricting access to abortion infringes on the reproductive rights and bodily autonomy of individuals. A group of medical professionals is hesitant about providing abortion services, as they face potential legal consequences and social backlash if they do so, and they have the option of conscientious objection. Argue your position regarding whether these medical professionals should or should not provide services.

Concluding Remarks

While there is no specific treaty explicitly referring to human rights to sexual and reproductive health, these rights are firmly embedded in the existing human rights framework. Nonetheless, the SRHR agenda remains unfinished, with significant disparities in sexual and reproductive health outcomes and access to comprehensive sexual and reproductive health services, in particular for girls, women and gender-diverse individuals.

This chapter argues that, if we consider it a primary task of our health systems to enable all individuals to attain "the highest attainable standard of health", significant challenges arise for those who are "othered" or marginalised due to their intersecting social positions in relation to structural systems of oppression. These individuals must be seen, understood, treated and cared for within a system not designed around their needs, experiences and knowledge. Navigating a social and health system influenced by gendered stereotypes often considered "normal" perpetuates pathways to poor health and violations of human rights, with the resulting prejudice and discrimination frequently going unnoticed.

Gender systems, including socially constructed norms and roles, as well as structural discrimination, are often misunderstood, overlooked and disregarded in research, health care systems and the delivery of health care. The various ways in which blindness to such gender systems manifests itself in (sexual and reproductive) health should be better understood and recognised as violations of human rights. By examining othering and compounded forms of discrimination, valuable lessons can be drawn for strategies to address health inequities in sexual and reproductive health and beyond.

Questions for Discussion

- Discuss the role that religious beliefs and/or cultural practices can play in the promotion of sexual and reproductive rights.
- Discuss why and how men should be involved in sexual and reproductive health programmes.
- Discuss how the right to life applies to sexual and reproductive rights.
- Discuss how the principle of non-discrimination applies to sexual and reproductive rights.
- Discuss how gender stereotyping can undermine SRHR.

Notes

1 The gender system is a network of interlinked domains – including family, community, institutions, and policies – that governs the distribution of power and the formation, reinforcement, and enforcement of gender norms. This system intersects with other axes of power and privilege, positioning individuals in various social hierarchies (Heise et al., 2019).
2 Existentialism is a philosophical movement which prioritises individual freedom, as well as responsibility and subjectivity.

References

Adami, R. (2018). *Women and the universal declaration of human rights*. Routledge.

Barnett, J. P., Maticka-Tyndale, E., & Kenya, T. (2016). Stigma as social control: Gender-based violence stigma, life chances, and moral order in Kenya. *Social Problems, 63*(3), 447–462.

Beal, F. M. (1969). *Double jeopardy: To be Black and female* (Vol. 1). Third World Women's Alliance. http://www.hartford-hwp.com/archives/45a/196.html

Beery, A. K., & Zucker, I. (2011). Sex bias in neuroscience and biomedical research. *Neuroscience & Biobehavioral Reviews, 35*(3), 565–572.

Berro Pizzarossa, L. (2018). Here to stay: The evolution of sexual and reproductive health and rights in international human rights law. *Laws, 7*(3), 29.

Bougie, O., Yap, M. I., Sikora, L., Flaxman, T., & Singh, S. (2019). Influence of race/ethnicity on prevalence and presentation of endometriosis: A systematic review and meta-analysis. *BJOG: An International Journal of Obstetrics & Gynaecology, 126*(9), 1104–1115.

Braveman, P., & Gruskin, S. (2003). Defining equity in health. *Journal of Epidemiology & Community Health, 57*(4), 254–258.

Collins, P. H. (1990). *Black feminist thought: Knowledge, consciousness, and the politics of empowerment*. Routledge.

Collins, P. H., & Bilge, S. (2016). *Intersectionality*. Polity Press.

Combahee River Collective. (1977). *The Combahee River Collective Statement*. Combahee River Collective.

Cook, R. J., & Cusack, S. (2010). *Gender stereotyping: Transnational legal perspectives*. University of Pennsylvania Press.

Courtenay, W. H. (2000). Constructions of masculinity and their influence on men's well-being: A theory of gender and health. *Social Science & Medicine, 50*(10), 1385–1401.

Crenshaw, K. (1989). Demarginalizing the intersection of race and sex: A Black feminist critique of antidiscrimination doctrine, feminist theory and antiracist politics. *University of Chicago Legal Forum, 1*, 139–167.

Cusack, S. (2013). Gender stereotyping as a human rights violation. *United Nations Human Rights, Office of the High Commissioner*, 13–30.

de Beauvoir, S. (2010). *The second sex*. Vintage Books.

de Vries, S. T., Denig, P., Ekhart, C., Burgers, J. S., Kleefstra, N., Mol, P. G., & van Puijenbroek, E. P. (2019). Sex differences in adverse drug reactions reported to the national pharmacovigilance centre in the Netherlands: An explorative observational study. *British Journal of Clinical Pharmacology*, 85(7), 1507–1515.

Dovidio, J. F., Hewstone, M., Glick, P., & Esses, V. M. (2010). Prejudice, stereotyping and discrimination: Theoretical and empirical overview. In J. F. Dovidio, M. Hewstone, P. Glick and V. M. Esses (Eds.), *Prejudice, Stereotyping and Discrimination* (pp. 3–28). Sage publications.

Green, C. R., Anderson, K. O., Baker, T. A., Campbell, L. C., Decker, S., Fillingim, R. B., Kalauokalani, D. A., Lasch, K. E., Myers, C., Tait, R. C., Todd, K. H., & Vallerand, A. H. (2003). The unequal burden of pain: Confronting racial and ethnic disparities in pain. *Pain Medicine*, 4(3), 277–294.

Hankivsky, O. (2012). Women's health, men's health, and gender and health: Implications of intersectionality. *Social Science & Medicine*, 74(11), 1712–1720.

Heise, L., Greene, M. E., Opper, N., Stavropoulou, M., Harper, C., Nascimento, M., Zewdie, D., Darmstadt, G. L., Greene, M., Hawkes, S. J., Henry, S., Heymann, J., Klugman, J., Levine, R., Raj, A., & Gupta, G. R. (2019). Gender inequality and restrictive gender norms: Framing the challenges to health. *The Lancet*, 393(10189), 2440–2454.

Hilton, J. L., & Von Hippel, W. (1996). Stereotypes. *Annual Review of Psychology*, 47(1), 237–271.

Jaffee, K. D., Shires, D. A., & Stroumsa, D. (2016). Discrimination and delayed health care among transgender women and men: Implications for improving medical education and health care delivery. *Medical Care*, 54(11), 1010–1016.

Kocas, H. D., Rubin, L. R., & Lobel, M. (2023). Stigma and mental health in endometriosis. *European Journal of Obstetrics & Gynecology and Reproductive Biology*, X, 100228.

Lane, S., Ayeb-Karlsson, S., & Shahvisi, A. (2021). Impacts of the global gag rule on sexual and reproductive health and rights in the Global South: A scoping review. *Global Public Health*, 16(12), 1804–1819.

Lyons, A. C. (2009). Masculinities, femininities, behaviour and health. *Social and Personality Psychology Compass*, 3(4), 394–412.

Maier, M., Samari, G., Ostrowski, J., Bencomo, C., & McGovern, T. (2021). "Scrambling to figure out what to do": A mixed method analysis of COVID-19's impact on sexual and reproductive health and rights in the United States. *BMJ Sexual & Reproductive Health*, 47(4), e16.

Manian, M. (2009). The irrational woman: Informed consent and abortion decision-making. *Duke Journal of Gender Law & Policy*, 16, 223.

Matías-González, Y., Sánchez-Galarza, A. N., Flores-Caldera, I., & Rivera-Segarra, E. (2021). "Es que tú eres una changa": Stigma experiences among Latina women living with endometriosis. *Journal of Psychosomatic Obstetrics & Gynecology*, 42(1), 67–74.

McGovern, T. (1997). Barriers to the inclusion of women in research and clinical trials. In N. Goldstein & J. L. Manlowe (Eds.), *The gender politics of HIV/AIDS in women: Perspectives on the pandemic in the United States* (pp. 43–62). New York University Press.

National Academies of Sciences, Engineering, and Medicine. (2018). *The safety and quality of abortion care in the United States*. The National Academies Press.

O'Connell, C., & Zampas, C. (2018). The human rights impact of gender stereotyping in the context of reproductive health care. *International Journal of Gynaecology & Obstetrics*, 144(1), 116–121.

Ojikutu, B. O., Pathak, S., Srithanaviboonchai, K., Limbada, M., Friedman, R., Li, S., Mimiaga, M. J., Mayer, K. H., Safren, S. A., & HIV Prevention Trials Network Team. (2016). Community cultural norms, stigma and disclosure to sexual partners among women living with HIV in Thailand, Brazil and Zambia (HPTN 063). *PLOS One*, 11(5), e0153600.

Parekh, A., Fadiran, E. O., Uhl, K., & Throckmorton, D. C. (2011). Adverse effects in women: Implications for drug development and regulatory policies. *Expert Review of Clinical Pharmacology*, 4(4), 453–466.

Pattyn, E., Verhaeghe, M., & Bracke, P. (2015). The gender gap in mental health service use. *Social Psychiatry and Psychiatric Epidemiology, 50*, 1089–1095.

Phillips, S. P., & Hamberg, K. (2016). Doubly blind: A systematic review of gender in randomised controlled trials. *Global Health Action, 9*(1), 29597.

Prentice, D. A., & Carranza, E. (2002). What women and men should be, shouldn't be, are allowed to be, and don't have to be: The contents of prescriptive gender stereotypes. *Psychology of Women Quarterly, 26*(4), 269–281.

Raday, F. (2007). Culture, religion, and CEDAW's article 5(a). In H. B. Schöpp-Schilling & C. Flinterman (Eds.), *The circle of empowerment: Twenty-five years of the UN committee on the elimination of discrimination against women* (pp. 68–85). The Feminist Press.

Runnels, V., Tudiver, S., Doull, M., & Boscoe, M. (2014). The challenges of including sex/gender analysis in systematic reviews: A qualitative survey. *Systematic Reviews, 3*, 1–10.

Seear, K. (2009). The etiquette of endometriosis: Stigmatisation, menstrual concealment and the diagnostic delay. *Social Science & Medicine, 69*(8), 1220–1227.

Singh, L., Abbas, S. M., Roberts, B., Thompson, N., & Singh, N. S. (2023). A systematic review of the indirect impacts of COVID-19 on sexual and reproductive health services and outcomes in humanitarian settings. *BMJ Global Health, 8*(11), e013477.

Stangor, C. (2009). The study of stereotyping, prejudice, and discrimination within social psychology. In T. D. Nelson (Ed.), *Handbook of prejudice, stereotyping and discrimination.* Psychology Press.

Starrs, A. M., & Anderson, R. (2016). Definitions and debates: Sexual health and sexual rights. *The Brown Journal of World Affairs, 22*(2), 7–23.

Starrs, A. M., Ezeh, A. C., Barker, G., Basu, A., Bertrand, J. T., Blum, R., Coll-Seck, A. M., Grover, A., Laski, L., Roa, M., Sathar, Z. A., Say, L., Serour, G. I., Singh, S., Stenberg, K., Temmerman, M., Biddlecom, A., Popinchalk, A., Summers, C., . . . & Ashford, L. S. (2018). Accelerate progress—sexual and reproductive health and rights for all: Report of the Guttmacher–Lancet Commission. *The Lancet, 391*(10140), 2642–2692.

Travis, C. B., Howerton, D. M., & Szymanski, D. M. (2012). Risk, uncertainty, and gender stereotypes in healthcare decisions. *Women & Therapy, 35*(3–4), 207–220.

UN. (1948). *Universal Declaration of Human Rights.* https://www.un.org/en/about-us/universal-declaration-of-human-rights

UN. (n.d.). *Vienna declaration and programme of action.* https://www.ohchr.org/en/instruments-mechanisms/instruments/vienna-declaration-and-programme-action

UNICEF. (2023). *Sexual and reproductive health.* https://data.unicef.org/topic/gender/sexual-and-reproductive-health/

UN Women. (1995). *Beijing declaration and platform for action.* https://www.un.org/womenwatch/daw/beijing/platform/

Van Eerdewijk, A., Kamunyu, M., Nyirinkindi, L., Sow, R., Visser, M. J., & Lodenstein, E. (2018). *The state of African women report.* KIT Royal Tropical Institute.

Whiteford, L. M., & Gonzalez, L. (1995). Stigma: The hidden burden of infertility. *Social Science & Medicine, 40*(1), 27–36.

WHO. (2009). *Women and health: Today's evidence tomorrow's agenda.* World Health Organization.

WHO. (2014). *Eliminating forced, coercive and otherwise involuntary sterilization: An interagency statement, OHCHR, UN Women, UNAIDS, UNDP, UNFPA, UNICEF and WHO.* World Health Organisation. https://iris.who.int/handle/10665/112848

WHO. (2023a). *Adolescent and young adult health.* https://www.who.int/news-room/fact-sheets/detail/adolescents-health-risks-and-solutions

WHO. (2023b). *WHO model list of essential medicines.* https://www.who.int/publications/i/item/WHO-MHP-HPS-EML-2023.02

WHO. (2024a). *Maternal mortality.* https://www.who.int/news-room/fact-sheets/detail/maternal-mortality

WHO. (2024b). *Adolescent pregnancy.* https://www.who.int/news-room/fact-sheets/detail/adolescent-pregnancy

WHO. (2024c). *Violence against women.* https://www.who.int/news-room/fact-sheets/detail/violence-against-women

WHO. (2024d). *Abortion.* https://www.who.int/news-room/fact-sheets/detail/abortion

WHO. (n.d.a). *Constitution.* https://www.who.int/about/accountability/governance/constitution

WHO. (n.d.b). *Gender and health.* https://www.who.int/health-topics/gender#tab=tab_1

WHO, UNICEF, United Nations Population Fund, & The World Bank. (2023). *Trends in maternal mortality: 2000 to 2020.* World Health Organization.

Yang, L. H., Poku, O. B., Misra, S., Mehta, H. T., Rampa, S., Eisenberg, M. M., Yang, L. S., Dai Cao, T. X., Blank, L. I., Becker, T. D., Link, B. G., Entaile, P., Opondo, P. R., Arscott-Mills, T., Ho-Foster, A. R., & Blank, M. B. (2021). Stigma, structural vulnerability, and "what matters most" among women living with HIV in Botswana, 2017. *American Journal of Public Health, 111*(7), 1309–1317.

Zhang, L., Losin, E. A. R., Ashar, Y. K., Koban, L., & Wager, T. D. (2021). Gender biases in estimation of others' pain. *The Journal of Pain, 22*(9), 1048–1059.

For Further Reading

Cicero, E. C., Reisner, S. L., Silva, S. G., Merwin, E. I., & Humphreys, J. C. (2019). Health care experiences of transgender adults: An integrated mixed research literature review. *Advances in Nursing Science, 42*(2), 123–138.

Corliss. (2022). *The heart disease gender gap: Social and cultural factors may help explain why women don't fare as well as men when it comes to treating coronary artery disease.* Harvard Health Publishing. https://www.health.harvard.edu/heart-health/the-heart-disease-gender-gap

de Beauvoir, S. (2010). *The second sex.* Vintage Books.

Miron-Shatz, T., Ormianer, M., Rabinowitz, J., Hanoch, Y., & Tsafrir, A. (2020). Physician experience is associated with greater underestimation of patient pain. *Patient Education and Counseling, 103*(2), 405–409.

Nichols, F. H. (2000). History of the women's health movement in the 20th century. *Journal of Obstetric, Gynecologic, & Neonatal Nursing, 29*(1), 56–64.

Samulowitz, A., Gremyr, I., Eriksson, E., & Hensing, G. (2018). "Brave men" and "emotional women": A theory-guided literature review on gender bias in health care and gendered norms towards patients with chronic pain. *Pain Research and Management, 2018*(1), 6358624.

WHO. *Human reproduction programme: Fifty years of achievement.* https://hrp50.srhr.org/

Disability and Human Rights

Mitzi M. Waltz

Introduction

Typically, about 15% of a country's population is comprised of disabled people (WHO & World Bank, 2011). This percentage often surprises people, but it is actually a conservative estimate. Far more people struggle with chronic ill health, mental health problems, learning difficulties, addiction, impairment due to injury and congenital conditions than those who have not been touched by these issues might think. Impairments can be physical (for example, cerebral palsy), sensory (for example, visual or hearing impairments), intellectual or psychosocial (for example, mental health difficulties or addiction). Chronic illness due to any cause is also a form of impairment.

When a person with an *impairment* or difference encounters societal, attitudinal or physical barriers that prevent them from full participation in society, their condition becomes a *disability*. In other words, while impairments are a fact of life, disablement is a process based on societal choices.

In low- and middle-income countries (LMICs), the percentage of persons with an impairment is often considerably higher. This is because the inhabitants of these countries are disproportionally affected by the disabling impacts of war, interpersonal violence, disease, work-related injury and poverty. For example, Rwanda has higher rates of disability than many other countries: as high as almost 20% in some districts (M'kumbuzi et al., 2013).

That said, high-income countries (HIC) often make societal choices that exclude – and therefore disable – larger categories of people based on tightening definitions of "normalcy". To give an example of how that works, in a traditional agrarian economy, a person with intelligence within the lower range or a learning difficulty like dyslexia can have a societal role that is as highly valued as anyone else's. In an economy where workers are expected to be highly educated, people with lower intellectual ability or learning disabilities are excluded and devalued: a difference is turned into a disability.

DOI: 10.4324/9781003408765-9

The social and economic exclusion of people with disabilities is complex as well as pervasive. It relies on definitions of "normalcy" that are culture-bound. These definitions can be based on religious beliefs, societal fears and prejudices, or beliefs that appeal to scientific knowledge. But, however distinctions are made between disabled and non-disabled, included or excluded, the fact remains: impairment and difference are *not* abnormal. While we all hope to achieve optimal health and function, this is not possible for many people. Human bodies and minds are diverse. In addition, almost all people will experience disability at some point in their life, especially as they get older.

Learning Objectives

After studying this chapter you will be able to:

- Understand the scope and nature of typical impairments and differences that can lead to disability
- Understand how people with impairments can become disabled
- Understand how the human rights of people with disability have historically been limited
- Discuss how disability intersects with other categories, such as sex, gender, "race", and socioeconomic status
- Discuss how to mainstream disability in development activities
- Discuss the social rights of persons with disabilities within the larger framework of human rights

Key Human Rights Frameworks

It is important to understand that, historically, many categories of disabled people have not been seen as having the same human rights as others. For example, people with intellectual difficulties have at times not been counted as "human". This has been demonstrated in many different ways. Currently and in the past, some people with an impairment have faced murder, violence, incarceration, institutionalisation, sterilisation, banishment, segregation and removal of their legal rights to make decisions, manage their own money, have a family or vote. Discrimination has been written into national laws and enforced by the state. Addressing these blatantly harmful and discriminatory policies has been the first target of human rights approaches to disability, but full inclusion of disabled people in society requires removal of all barriers to participation. Moving towards these goals has required progressive change to human rights frameworks.

The UDHR (1948) established social rights as part of human rights for the first time. However, because it was truly the first global agreement on human rights, securing social rights tended to take a back seat to issues like preventing torture that were very current at the end of World War II, when the declaration was written.

The ICESCR (1966) tried to move forward this wider human rights agenda. Again, disabled people were not at the forefront of this effort. Although they were clearly covered by both the Declaration and the Covenant, they did not usually benefit from either one when it came to discrimination and maltreatment based on disability.

In 1971, the Declaration on the Rights of Mentally Retarded Persons declared that individuals with intellectual disabilities should have equal human rights to other people, including the right to live with their families rather than in institutions, and the right to not be harmed or exploited. This provides examples of *positive rights* – the right to do something – and *negative rights* – the right to not be harmed by something or to not be forced to do something.

The 1971 Declaration started the process towards a disability-specific human rights act. Finally, the UN recognised that violations of human rights based on disability were pervasive internationally, and were not being addressed sufficiently by "generic" human rights laws and policies. In tandem with specific actions for women, children, migrants and Indigenous people, the UN Convention on the Rights of Persons with Disabilities (CRPD) was created in 2006 to specify human rights in relation to the situation of disabled people and their unique needs (UN, 2020). The UN CRPD was developed with a great deal of input from Disabled People's Organisations (DPOs): it was not just an idea developed at an elite level by experts, but resulted from a growing call from disabled people themselves.

The Netherlands was one of the last major countries to sign and ratify the UN CRPD, in 2016. By ratifying this agreement, a country agrees to align its national laws and policies with the UN CRPD. In the Netherlands, this has been a lengthy process, and it is not yet complete. Also, although cases based on the UN CRPD can be brought to a national human rights body, the College van de Rechten van de Mens, there is no enforcement mechanism even when a case of discrimination or human rights violation is found.

In most countries, there is still a long way to go. The United States, for example, has signed but not ratified the UN CRPD, meaning it is not yet bound to uphold the obligations listed in it. Some other countries that have both signed and ratified have either not changed discriminatory legislation and practices, or have been very slow to act despite their agreement on paper.

In addition to these international human rights actions, there have been a number of important regional and national actions regarding the human rights of disabled people. These include, for example, the African Charter on Human and Peoples' Rights (1981), the ASEAN Enabling Masterplan (2025), the Disability Discrimination Act in the UK (DDA, 1992), the Individuals with Disabilities Education Act (IDEA, 1975) and the Americans with Disabilities Act (ADA, 1990) in the US, the Brazilian Inclusion Law (2015) and the European Accessibility Act (2015).

There are often conflicts between the vision of universal human rights and laws and policies that try to lay out the rights of – or protections for – groups of people who are seen as specifically vulnerable. This is also true when it comes to the rights of people with disabilities. For example, the African Charter on Human and Peoples' Rights mentions disabled people specifically as follows:

> the aged and disabled shall also have the right to special measures of protection in keeping with their physical and/or moral needs.

There can be conflicts between individual rights and calls for protection, for example in situations such as guardianship, and unravelling these can be complex.

Impairment and Disability

At the beginning of this chapter, I used two words that actually have quite different meanings: *impairment* and *disability*. This distinction is based on a new way of looking at disability, which arose from disabled people's organisations in the UK in the 1980s: the *social model of disability* (Barnes & Mercer, 2004). Prior to this innovation, the assumed basis for discussing disability issues was what is now known as the "medical model" of disability. The social and medical models of disability start from very different key premises, and this decision to rely on one model or the other dictates what solutions are seen as valid.

The medical model looks at human difference or impairment as a property of individual bodies. The "problem" of disability, in this case, is seen as being within the disabled person, and the solutions are to be found in medical treatment and care by others. If the person cannot be "fixed", the state or charity may or may not accept responsibility to provide practical help or support.

The social model separates impairment – medical or functional facts about a person's body, health or ability – from their societal position. Of course, ill health and impairment are still a target for medical intervention. But the social circumstances that surround people with impairments and differences, such as inaccessible housing, job discrimination and negative attitudes, are seen as turning these into a disability. In this model, the "problem" of disability is a social one and can be best addressed through social change that prevents exclusion and promotes inclusion.

Two illustrations are often used to explain the difference:

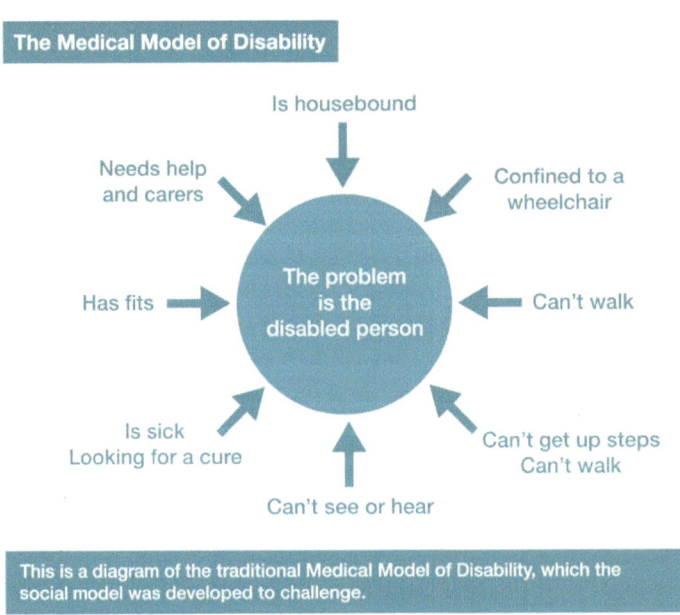

Figure 6.1a The Medical Model of Disability

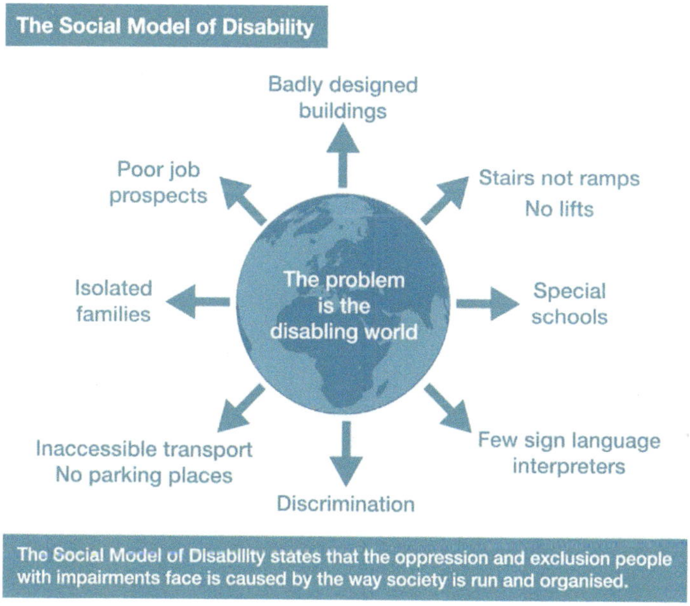

The Social Model of Disability

Badly designed
buildings

Poor job
prospects

Stairs not ramps
No lifts

Isolated
families

The problem
is the
disabling world

Special
schools

Inaccessible transport
No parking places

Few sign language
interpreters

Discrimination

The Social Model of Disability states that the oppression and exclusion people
with impairments face is caused by the way society is run and organised.

Figure 6.1b The Social Model of Disability

Here's a way of looking at it that shows why the social model aligns better with a human rights approach to disability:

Table 6.1 Medical Model and Social Model

	Medical model	*Social model*
Problem	The problem is the person with the impairment	The problem is in society/environment
	A person with an impairment is broken or sick	A person with a disability faces physical and/or social barriers
	Disability is located in the body of the person with an impairment	Attitudes, perceptions and the physical environment cause disability
Solution/power	A person with a disability requires healing/curing	Barriers in the environment and society need to be removed
	Health and social care professionals and/or individuals are responsible	Governments and societies are responsible
	Non-disabled people make choices, control policy and services	People with disabilities make their own choices, control policy and services
	Governments and professionals may avoid responsibilities	Focus on participation rather than treatment: governments and professionals should focus on supports and societal changes that enable it

Both the social model and the medical model have informed an important tool used to look at disability in the global health context: the International Classification of Functioning, Disability and Health, better known as the ICF framework (WHO, 2023). This is important because, to access human rights that are specific to a category, people need to be recognised as belonging to that category. If someone is not recognised as disabled, they cannot claim rights based on that status. The ICF is an imperfect framework, but because it acknowledges that both medical facts and societal choices can impact people's lives, it can be used to show how denial of human rights is part of the process of disablement.

Disability: An Intersectional Approach

Disabled people are more than just their disability label. They have personalities, individual hopes and dreams; they are enmeshed in families and cultures. Disability also does not stand alone when it comes to conveying disadvantage: there are many intersections between disability and age, sex, gender, "race" and socioeconomic status, and these can combine to increase or decrease disadvantage (also see Chapter 5).

Frequently, attribution of disability has been used to devalue specific groups. Examples of this are the attribution of "low IQ" to Black people and the inclusion of homosexuality in the *Diagnostic and Statistical Manual* of the American Psychiatric Association (Longmore & Umansky, 2001). In several countries, including the former Soviet Union, political dissidents have been identified as "mentally ill", allowing the state to use laws removing the civil rights of people with mental illness to lock them up without a trial (van Voren, 2010). Historically, women have been depicted as "the weaker sex", with males portrayed as "normal" (as introduced in Chapter 5). As with political dissidents, women who choose to step outside of expected social roles have sometimes been defined as "mentally ill" and drugged or incarcerated. Migrants and refugees are often connected with fear of "contagion": during the COVID-19 pandemic, the US has used this as an excuse for deporting asylum seekers at its southern border, citing fear that they would bring COVID-19 into the US. Concepts of racial superiority, male dominance and "purity" are closely tied to the concept of the "normal" person that is used to define disability, and attribution of disability to others is often used to define the "normal" person through false comparisons.

One way in which the human rights of disabled people have been violated is the practice of *eugenics*: the pseudoscience of improving the human race through selective breeding (and, in some cases, outright murder). In the early 1900s, these ideas became very popular in Europe and the US. They drove institutionalisation of vast numbers of disabled people. Many were sterilised as well. Hitler took these ideas to the extreme: the Holocaust actually began with the murder of disabled people in institutions, long before the concentration camps were set up. Depicting Jews, Gypsies and homosexuals as disease-ridden burdens on the state was also one of the methods the Nazis used to convince others to accept that they should be killed.

Today, eugenics seems to be making a comeback. In the UK, prime minister Boris Johnson hired a special advisor, Dominic Cummings, who until his fall from grace during the COVID-19 epidemic was widely seen as the untouchable "power behind the throne". Cummings has openly stated that he believes intelligence is mostly inherited and more common among the wealthy upper classes, and education is wasted on the less intelligent (and therefore on the poor) (Cummings, 2013). This view suggests that societal elites are born to rule, and others are born to serve. In the US, former president Trump frequently referred to "good genes" that convey superiority (Currell, 2019). In the Netherlands, the politician Thierry Baudet has championed eugenics and met with racist theorists who claim that non-white people are intellectually inferior (Tokmetzis et al., 2017). Eugenic beliefs and actions continue to have adherents in LMICs as well (e.g., Chung, 2014; Wilson, 2018).

Upholding human rights for all requires rejecting these damaging, demeaning and scientifically false beliefs. When you see disability (especially but not only intellectual inferiority) attributed to a group or type of person, pay close attention: because disabled people have historically been dehumanised, this is an effort to make someone appear to be less than human and therefore to place them as lacking full human rights.

Example: Dalits and Disability in India

In India, the caste system has existed for a long time. Ideas about caste began in notions of ritual purity: who is fit to serve as a priest in the temple. This concept is also one of the roots of ideas about "purity" that underlie ideas about disability in Western culture, where they derive from Christianity, Judaism and Greco-Roman religious practices. In India, caste rules became solidified when the Mughal empire fell, and the British colonialists took over. Under British rule, caste and religion were used as criteria for offering or denying work and favours.

Although caste distinctions were legally banned in the Indian constitution of 1948, the caste system continues to exist and determines many aspects of people's lives. Caste rules include residential and occupational segregation, and rules on intermarriage and social interactions, amongst other behaviours.

Ideas about disability were and are instrumental in forming ideas about caste. Low-caste people such as the Dalits ("untouchables") are portrayed by upper-caste people as being born less able and less intelligent, or only suited for certain kinds of menial work. And caste itself contributes to disability. For example, despite affirmative action programmes, Dalits are generally very poor and so are more likely to suffer from malnutrition, accidents, violence and untreated illness – all factors that contribute to a higher rate of disability in this population (Pal, 2010).

Gobinda Pal (2010) notes that

The interface of "caste" and "disability" on the life of Dalits remains stubbornly in place. It can strongly reinforce underlying disadvantages bearing significant negative consequences on the lives of Dalits with disabilities. Physical limitations coupled with Dalit identity are likely to put them "at greater risk".

Consider this in light of the disability-poverty cycle:

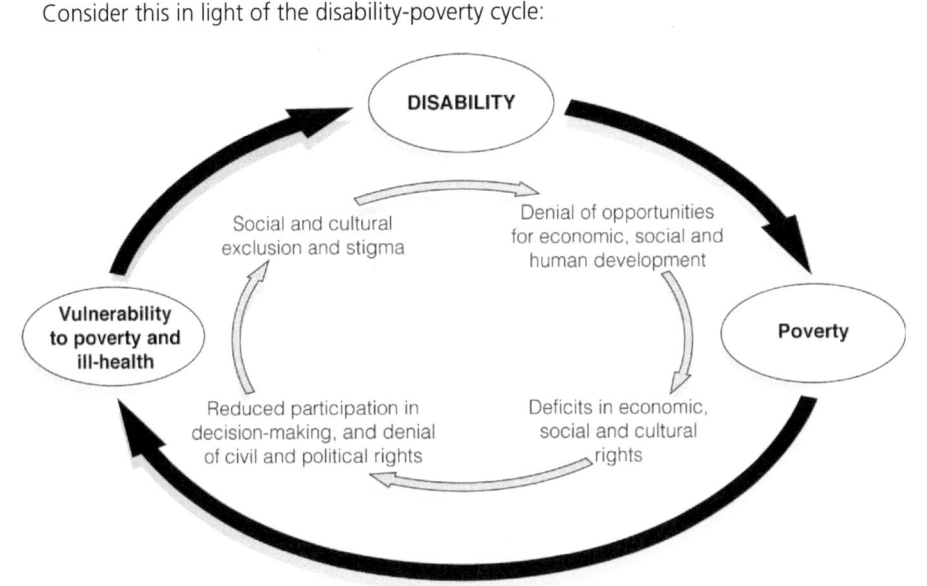

Figure 6.2 Disability–poverty Vulnerability Cycle

Questions for Discussion

■ How do notions of caste, "race" and "purity" interact with disablement to produce disadvantage in India?

■ Can you think of ways that a similar process takes place in your own country, perhaps with intersections among socioeconomic status, "race", sexuality, gender and/or migrant status and disability?

Example: Disability and Old Age

As noted at the beginning of this chapter, almost everyone who reaches old age will eventually experience physical and/or mental impairment. In some societies, older people hold a privileged position in society. When they acquire age-related impairments, they may also hold a privileged position in comparison to other disabled people. There may be less stigma attached to impairments when they are associated with age, for example.

In some other societies, impairment can have tremendous negative consequences for older people. This can be as extreme as deprivation of liberty, meaning that the person loses the right to give or deny consent and is no longer allowed to decide where they will live or how they will spend their time. In some countries, older people with impairments face increased pressure to end their own lives through euthanasia.

Questions for Discussion

- In your own country, are older people with impairments viewed differently from younger disabled people? What is the difference, and why do you think this might be?

- Although it is common to paint notions of familial duty to care for older people as positive, familial care also has a negative side: it is mainly women who shoulder the burden of care for disabled adults and seniors. What impacts do you think these care duties have on the lives of women? Can you think of ways to organise care for disabled seniors other than familial care or institutionalisation?

Supporting and Ensuring the Human Rights of Disabled People

Development is typically understood as changes that improve the lives of people in LMICs. However, disabled people are sometimes negatively affected by development processes, such as population movement from the countryside to the city or higher educational requirements for work. They also already lack equal access to services and goods (Grills et al., 2017). Within HICs there are also populations who lack adequate access to human rights and societal goods, despite an overall higher standard of living. In Europe, the most prominent of these are Roma/Sinti/Traveller communities, Indigenous populations in the far north (e.g., the Sami), undocumented migrants and disabled people.

As already noted, typical societal barriers to human rights for disabled people include:

- Physical barriers, for example when someone cannot vote because the polling place or ballot is not accessible
- Stigma and discrimination, for example when, because of a stigmatised impairment, someone is not accepted as a teacher or medical professional, or when a qualified disabled person is passed over for a job in favour of a non-disabled person
- Segregation, for example when, to receive the care a physically disabled person needs, they are forced to live in a special "care village" or in a care home instead of a regular residence

Typical legal and policy barriers to human rights for disabled people include:

- Eugenic laws (e.g., forced sterilisation, euthanasia, forced segregation)
- Mental capacity laws and guardianship
- Discriminatory rules related to professional licensing or "fitness to work"

The root of many of these barriers is negative attitudes about people with disabilities. If lawmakers, voters, policymakers, decision-makers and employers did not often share these negative attitudes, these barriers would be hard for them to justify.

Solutions include removing negative measures – such as laws that exclude disabled people from full citizenship or place them in segregated settings – and enacting positive measures, such as taking actions to ensure disabled people can vote, marry, have children, have a voice and make choices.

Another important way of addressing the human rights of disabled people is called the capability approach (Trani, 2015). This framework for action states that freedom to attain well-being is a crucial moral good and that we need to consider what actual opportunities people have to do so. This can mean using development plans and actions to add to those capabilities: for example, providing skills training, making societal changes that open up access to land to grow food or involving disadvantaged people in decision-making about their lives. These processes should be designed to help disabled and other disadvantaged people to build human, social, psychological and societal capital and put it to use to benefit themselves and their communities.

The goal of such processes is sometimes called "just" development: development that ensures the benefits of change are widely distributed instead of flowing mainly to societal elites. For disabled people in particular, that can sometimes mean opting for the twin-track approach to development (Dadun et al., 2018): disabled people should be included in all development activities to make sure their needs are known and met, but there may also need to be some disability-specific activities, such as skills training and formation of Disabled Peoples Organisations that can advocate for their specific needs.

Social Rights and Disability

As discussed earlier, social rights are a subset of human rights, also known as social, economic and cultural rights. They include the right to adequate food and water, housing, education, work, health and participation in society. Access to food, water, shelter and health care are necessary to sustain life, whereas other social rights, such as the right to education, work and participation, allow people to be part of and contribute to society and also provide them with the means to obtain the other essentials. Other rights recognised in this category include the right to benefit from scientific discoveries, practice one's religion, speak one's own language, take part in one's own culture and join a trade union.

When it comes to the social rights to food, water and shelter, there is often a misconception that placing these as human rights means that everyone has a right to "free stuff". But social rights are actually about ensuring everyone has the right to access, create, grow, use or purchase necessities – except in emergencies, when governments (and the international community) do indeed have a duty to provide affected persons with the essentials to support life. In everyday life, these social rights are not just about having "just enough to prevent death", they include having access to food that is sufficient for good health, culturally appropriate and personally acceptable.

Even in HICs, where ensuring social rights are protected does not run up against significant financial barriers, people with disabilities are often particularly disadvantaged. They may face physical, societal and attitudinal barriers, as well as the financial barriers presented by the disability-poverty cycle you have just looked at. For example, where financial assistance is provided to help people access or adapt housing, the funds may be much lower than actual costs, and the total amount budgeted for all disabled people is limited, so only those seen as having the "most severe" disabilities are allowed help. This can force groups of disabled people into competition with each other and place individuals with disability in a position where they need to downplay their abilities or avoid paid employment just to obtain enough income to stay alive.

> **Textbox 6.1**
> **Case Study**
>
> Luiz is a 27-year-old from Venezuela who has come to the Netherlands due to political upheaval in his native country. An armed gang has attacked his village, targeting young men. If the young men will not join their militia group, they kill them. Luiz luckily escaped his village and the country, and he has been accepted as a refugee. Now he needs to get through the citizenship ("inburgering") process (language and citizenship education) so that he will be allowed to live and work here.
>
> Luiz never did well in school and can barely read or write. The teacher of his course notices that Luiz is having more trouble than the others, and refers him for a dyslexia assessment. After the assessment, Luiz knows that he has something called dyslexia, and this may well be why school was so difficult when he was younger.
>
> However, the citizenship requirements are not very flexible: he must attain a certificate based on passing several written language tests (in Dutch) and a written Dutch culture test. He must submit a written job-seeking portfolio and attend an interview about employment. There is a time limit: if he cannot achieve all these milestones in time, he will not be allowed to stay.
>
> As he tries to complete his employment portfolio, Luiz runs into another problem. He used to work as an auto mechanic. In Venezuela, he did not need any formal qualification for this. He has a natural ability with diagnosing and fixing engine problems – whether it's a lawnmower or an Audi – and years of hands-on experience. But in the Netherlands, auto mechanics need to complete a course and be certified to work on various models. Luiz looks at the course. He would have to go to school for 2–3 years, studying with mostly teenagers. There would be a lot of written work, in Dutch. He feels very discouraged about the prospect of ever working on cars again, and decides to complete the work portfolio with examples about doing warehouse work instead.
>
> **Questions for Discussion:**
>
> ■ Where can you locate disabling barriers in the story of Luiz? In what ways are these barriers intersectional (not just about disability)?
> ■ What are some ways that society could respond to these barriers to help Luiz reach his full potential and participate fully in society?
> ■ Why does the social model of disability offer a more useful framework for considering the impact of Luiz's disability and a human rights-based approach for addressing it?

Questions for Discussion

Working in small groups, we will focus on the right to food in a Dutch context, using the article from M. Waltz et al. (2018) (see reference list) as a basis for the discussion.

■ One group of students will devise a policy for food banks that ensures people with disabilities have access to adequate food. Barriers are described in the article – students in this group will need to identify the barriers and come up with a policy that would address these, with attention to the definition presented in *ICESCR*

General Comment No. 12: The Right to Adequate Food (Art. 11) (OHCRH, 1999).

■ Another group of students will devise a policy regarding food in residential homes that ensures people with disabilities who live in congregate settings have access to adequate food. Barriers are described in the article – students will need to identify them and come up with a policy that would address these, with attention to the definition presented in *ICESCR General Comment No. 12: The Right to Adequate Food* (Art. 11).

■ If there is a need for a third group of students due to numbers, that group can consider what innovative measures could be put in place to ensure greater food security for disabled people, beyond cash benefits and food banks. Choose one innovative approach and prepare a policy brief for a city or national government to convince policymakers about why it should be implemented. Pay attention to attention to the definition of the right to food presented in *ICESCR General Comment No. 12: The Right to Adequate Food* (Art. 11).

Concluding Remarks

Understanding the distinction between impairment and disability reveals the importance of societal change in addressing disability. The medical model's focus on individual deficits contrasts with the social model's emphasis on removing societal barriers and promoting inclusion. Disability intersects with other social categories such as age, gender, race and socioeconomic status, often compounding the disadvantages faced by individuals. Addressing these intersections is essential for ensuring human rights.

The historical and ongoing struggles for the human rights of disabled people highlight the progress made and the challenges that remain. The establishment of key human rights frameworks, such as the CRPD, marks significant milestones in recognising and addressing the rights of disabled people. However, the implementation and enforcement of these frameworks continue to require sustained effort and commitment, and the inclusion of disabled people in development processes is often limited. As we move forward, it is imperative to continue advocating for the removal of societal barriers, challenging negative attitudes and promoting inclusive policies and systems that uphold human rights.

Questions for Discussion

■ What conflicts can you see between the idea of protecting disabled people and ensuring that disabled people have full human rights?

■ Do disability benefit programmes in your country help recipients to build human, social, psychological and societal capital? If so, how? If not, why not? How could benefit programmes be designed to empower disabled people?

■ Read the article on the right to food in a Dutch context, using the article by M. Waltz et al. (2018) (see reference list).

    ■ Discuss how food banks can ensure that people with disabilities have access to adequate food. Take into account ICESCR General Comment No. 12: The Right to Adequate Food (Art. 11).

- Discuss how residential homes can ensure that people with disabilities who live in congregate settings have access to adequate food. Take into account ICESCR General Comment No. 12: The Right to Adequate Food (Art. 11).
- Why do you think social rights are the most difficult part of human rights to convince society to support and enact?
- Why is it important to avoid relying on charities to ensure social rights – why can that approach create hierarchies and new barriers for people with disabilities?

References

Barnes, C., & Mercer, G. (2004). Theorising and researching disability from a social model perspective. In C. Barnes & G. Mercer (Eds.), *Implementing the social model in disability theory and research*. The Disability Press.

Dadun, D., Peters, R. M., van Brakel, W. H., Bunders, J. G., Irwanto, I., & Regeer, B. J. (2018). Assessing the impact of the twin track socio-economic intervention on reducing leprosy-related stigma in Cirebon District, Indonesia. *International Journal of Environmental Research and Public Health*, 16(3), 349.

Chung, Y. J. (2014). Better science and better race?: Social Darwinism and Chinese eugenics. *Isis*, 105(4), 793–802. doi: 10.1086/679426

Cummings, D. (2013). Some thoughts on education and political priorities [online post, republished]. *The Guardian*, London. Online: https://www.theguardian.com/politics/interactive/2013/oct/11/dominic-cummings-michael-gove-thoughts-education-pdf

Currell, S. (2019) 'This may be the most dangerous thing Donald Trump believes': Eugenic populism and the American body politic. *Amerikastudien/American Studies*, 64(2), 291–302. http://www.jstor.org/stable/45390293

Grills, N., Singh, L., Pant, H., Varghese, J., Murthy, G. V. S., Hoq, M., & Marella, M. (2017). Access to services and barriers faced by people with disabilities: A quantitative survey. *Disability, CBR & Inclusive Development*, 28(2), 23.

Longmore, P., & Umansky, L. (2001). *The new disability history*. New York University Press.

M'kumbuzi, V. R. P., Sagahutu, J. B., Kagwiza, J., Urimubenshi, G., & Mostert-Wentzel, K. (2014). The emerging pattern of disability in Rwanda. *Disability and Rehabilitation*, 36(6), 472–478.

OHCRH. (1999). *CESCR general comment no. 12: The right to adequate food* (Art. 11). United Nations. https://www.refworld.org/pdfid/4538838c11.pdf

Pal, G. C. (2010). *Dalits with disabilities: The neglected dimension of social exclusion* (Indian Institute of Dalit Studies Working Power Series, IV(3)). Indian Institute of Dalit Studies. http://www.dalitstudies.org.in/wp/1003.pdf

Tokmetzis, D., l'Ami, D., & van Biezen, M. (2017). Thierry Baudet ontmoette in her geheim een Amerikaanse racist van alt-right. *De Correspondent*, 20 December. Online: https://decorrespondent.nl/7738/thierry-baudet-ontmoette-in-het-geheim-een-amerikaanse-racist-van-alt-right

Trani, J.-F., Bakhshi, P., Bellanca, N., Biggeri, M., & Marchetta, F. (2015). Disabilities through the capability approach lens: Implications for public policies. *Alter*, 5(3), 143–157.

UN. (2020). *Convention on the rights of persons with disabilities (CRPD)*. UN Department of Social and Economic Affairs. https://www.un.org/development/desa/disabilities/convention-on-the-rights-of-persons-with-disabilities.html

Van Voren, R. (2010). Political abuse of psychiatry – an historical overview. *Schizophrenia Bulletin*, 36(1), 33–35.

Waltz, M., Mol, T., Gittins, E., & Schippers, A. (2018). Disability, access to food and the UN CRPD: Navigating discourses of human rights in the Netherlands. *Social Inclusion*, 6(1), 51–60.

WHO. (2023). *International Classification of Functioning, Disability and Health (ICF)* [web site]. World Health Organization. https://www.who.int/standards/classifications/international-classification-of-functioning-disability-and-health

WHO & World Bank. (2011). *World report on disability*. World Health Organization. https://www.who.int/teams/noncommunicable-diseases/sensory-functions-disability-and-rehabilitation/world-report-on-disability

Wilson, K. (2018). For reproductive justice in an era of Gates and Modi: The violence of India's population policies. *Feminist Review, 119*(1), 89–105.

CHAPTER 7

Mental Health and Psychiatric Care

Miryam R. R. Holguín, Cees J. Hamelink and Tesania Velázquez

Introduction

The Special UN Rapporteur, in a report to the UN Human Rights Council (Forty-fourth session, 15 June–3 July 2020), welcomes the international recognition that there is no health without mental health and appreciates the different worldwide initiatives to advance all elements of global mental health: promotion, prevention, treatment, rehabilitation and recovery. However, the Rapporteur also emphasises that, despite promising trends, there remains a global failure of the status quo to address human rights violations in mental health care systems.

The WHO defines mental health as a "state of well-being in which every individual realises his or her own potential, can cope with the normal stresses of life, can work productively and fruitfully, and is able to make a contribution to her or his community". This definition implies that mental health is reliant on a wide array of factors that include, among others, physical health, the availability of adequate housing, just and favourable conditions for work and freedom from discrimination, all of which are enshrined in international human rights law.

The relationship between mental health and human rights has at least three parts. First, human rights violations such as torture and displacement negatively affect mental health. Second, mental health practices, such as coercive treatment practices, impact human rights. Third, the advancement of human rights benefits people's mental health conditions. There are clinical and economic reasons, as well as moral and legal obligations, to advance human rights in mental health care.

Learning Objectives
After studying this chapter you will be able to:

- Contribute to discussions about the state of mental health in the world
- Contribute to the future of rights-based mental health care

DOI: 10.4324/9781003408765-10

■ Discuss mental health care from the perspective of the Convention on the Rights of Persons with Disabilities (CRPD) and argue for or against an international convention on mental health care

The Factsheet

The WHO definition of health mentions mental well-being and recognises depression as the second most common of the world's common diseases. One in every eight people in the world lives with a mental disorder. In 2019, one in every eight people, 970 million people around the world, were living with a mental disorder, with anxiety and depressive disorders the most common. In 2020, the number of people living with anxiety and depressive disorders rose significantly because of the COVID-19 pandemic. Initial estimates show a 26% and 28% increase respectively for anxiety and major depressive disorders in just one year. While effective prevention and treatment options exist, most people with mental disorders do not have access to effective care. Mental illness affects nearly one in three individuals globally during their lifetime and nearly one in five in the past 12 months. Mental and substance abuse disorders were leading causes of disability and were responsible for 8.6 million years lost to premature death worldwide in 2010. The burden of these disorders increased by 37.6% from 1990 to 2010. The annual economic cost of mental illness globally has been estimated to be $2.5 trillion, with a projected increase to $6 trillion by 2030, more than half of the total costs for all non-communicable diseases. In the Netherlands one of four people suffers from mental disorders. In 2022, 2.5 million people took psychopharmaca, among them more than one million took anti-depressants and some 40,000 kids took a daily dose of Ritalin to deal with a problem diagnosed as ADHD.

In world politics, powerful leaders have been diagnosed with serious personality disorders. Examples are Lincoln, Roosevelt, Churchill, Chruchev: manic depressions. Hitler, Pol Pot, Stalin, Mao: megalomania. Nixon: paranoia, Johnson: bipolarity, Bush Jr: narcissism, Trump: pathological malignant narcissism. Yet, there is little recognition around the world of mental illnesses that usually have a low priority in national health policies. This is reflected in the allocation of resources and training facilities. In many countries, mental disorders are still a taboo issue. One third of UN members have no mental health policy at all. Only 100 member states have a mental health budget which is usually less than 1% of the overall health budget. Almost half of UN member states have no training facilities for mental health care.

Human rights violations in the mental health context remain significant throughout the world, including in high-, middle- and low-income countries. The prevalence of rights abuse cannot be explained by a mere lack of resources. In the relatively wealthy European region, for example, funds continue to be invested in the renovation and expansion of large-scale residential and psychiatric institutions. These sites perpetuate a vicious cycle of exclusion and despair. The rise elsewhere of involuntary psychiatric intervention in hospitals and homes also suggests that something is wrong. There are serious arguments by professionals who warn against a prohibition of forced treatment. They insist that the legal permission to treat individuals with serious mental health conditions involuntarily should be retained. Against these arguments there are the professionals who argue that the non-consensual imposition of mind- and body-altering drugs based on narrow conceptions of impairment, poorly evidenced claims about "risk" and "necessity" and a limited range of alternatives is incompatible with dignity and autonomy.

Historical Development

In the 19th century, the biomedical approach prevailed in psychiatry. The "scientific" ambitions of 19th-century psychiatry led to surgical interventions in the brains of disturbed people. In mental institutions, medical professionals applied lobotomy and would often enter the frontal brain with an ice-pick. Without any scientific evidence such lobotomies – and also electroshock and insulin shock therapies – were introduced. The great lobotomist Antonio Egas Moniz even got the Nobel Prize for the discovery of the therapeutic effect of lobotomy in 1949. For the father of modern psychiatry, Emil Kraepelin, it was clear that psychiatric disorder were disorders of the brain. There was and is, however, no scientific evidence that there is something in the brain that can explain psychiatric disorders. In the early 20th century a psychological approach emerged (with psychiatrists as Freud, Jung and Adler) that shifted the focus from organic deficiencies to psychological causes such as conflicts between the conscious and the unconscious that might cause neurosis, depression and anxiety. The mid-20th century saw the development of a critical social approach (with, among others, Ronald Laing) that defended that society is the cause of mental disorders. The most recent is the neurological approach that is convinced that it is all in the brain. This raises the question of whether we go back a hundred years to the biomedical model.

It looks like mental health and mental health care are entering in the early 21st century, the digital age, with the advent of online psychiatry, TikTok self-diagnoses and memes about suicidal thoughts on Instagram.

Cultural Perceptions of Mental Health

Mental health is a complex issue that can be affected by many different factors. Among them culture plays a significant role in shaping how people think and feel about their mental health. It is important to understand culture's role in mental health to create an inclusive and effective environment for mental health care. We should look at the role of family, religion, prevailing behavioural norms and cultural traditions. Every culture has a different way of looking at mental health. For many in the world, there still is an enormous stigma around mental health, and mental health issues are considered personal weaknesses, which makes it difficult to talk openly and to ask for help.

Culture can influence how people describe and feel about their symptoms. Cultural beliefs and values can affect how people see themselves and the world around them. In some cultures, it is more acceptable to express emotions openly, while in others emotional restraint is the norm. This can affect how people cope with stressful situations and how well they bounce back from setbacks. Some cultures may also emphasise individualism, while others may emphasise the importance of community and interdependence. This can affect views about ourselves and others. Depressive moods and anxiety disorders are found across all cultures. However, they tend to be expressed differently in different cultures. In Western cultures, anxiety is often experienced as fear or dread. In contrast, in Eastern cultures, it may be more likely to be experienced as physical symptoms such as heart palpitations or dizziness. In the West, mental disorders are often seen as medical conditions that need to be treated with medication or other medical interventions. But in many traditional cultures, mental health problems are seen as spiritual issues that need to be addressed through religious or shamanic rituals. An interesting example is provided by a study of Hisham Abu-Raiya (2015) who built a personality theory on the idea that, from an Islamic perspective, the human soul consists of divine and evil aspects, and he developed the Qur'an-Based Psychotherapy Model that aims to treat psychological problems by taming the evil side and empowering the divine side. We can also cite illustrations from Africa. One of these is the Meseron therapy, which means "I reject it". This was developed by clinical psychologist Alfred Awaritefe in Nigeria and aims to enable clients to use their resources to dissociate from undesirable situations, to become constructive and to "reject the negative and accept the positive" (Afolabi & Joy, 2014). Another African approach to psychotherapy is the Ubuntu therapy of South Africa origin which is based on a worldview that highlights collectiveness and interdependence and aims to solve clients' problems by addressing them in relation to the creator, other people and the self; it uses various techniques from dancing to storytelling (Van Dyk & Nefale, 2005).

As mental health providers across the world have to work with clients that are often from cultures other than their own, they need to explore and learn how differences in cultures have implications for mental health practice, ranging from the ways that people view health and illness to treatment-seeking patterns, the nature of the therapeutic relationship and issues of racism and discrimination. More work needs to be done in finding ways in which mental health care systems and their professionals can engage across cultures more equitably and sustainably. By and large, cultural factors have still not found a place in the prevailing biological perspectives on mental health and psychotherapy. A major reason behind this is the conception of a mental disorder as a biologically caused disease that follows universal processes. Western "enlightenment" assumptions about individuality, rationality, measurability and reductionism are driving the dominant model of mental health care. However, in Western societies psychiatrists have made the discovery that conceptions of schizophrenia in France differ from those in the UK. Fortunately, today there is more critical study and debate on the role of cultural factors in perceptions of the formation of mental disorders and the thinking on psychotherapy.

Mental Disorders

There are many different types of mental disorders. They may also be referred to as mental health conditions. This broad term covers mental states that are characterised by excessive anxiety, guilt, low self-esteem, hopelessness, the alternation of depressed moods with manic symptoms, delusions, eating disorders or post-traumatic stress disorders. All these states may result in a serious impairment in functioning or risks of self-harm. There are treatment options available, but most people in the world do not have access to effective mental health care.

The Problem of Diagnostics in Mental Health Care

For diagnostics in mental health care there is a diagnostic manual: the *Diagnostic and Statistical Manual of Mental Disorders* (DSM). The DSM lists criteria for the classification of mental disorders. It is widely used by health professionals, researchers, counsellors, psychologists and psychiatrists. For each disorder, there is a set of diagnostic criteria with specific symptoms that characterise the disorder. The DSM is published by the American Psychiatric Association (APA) and was originally published in 1952. The DSM is now in its fifth edition (DSM-5), and the DSM-5 was published in 2013.

There are two main interrelated criticisms of DSM-5: an unhealthy influence of the pharmaceutical industry on the revision process and an increasing tendency to "medicalise" patterns of behaviour and moods that may not considered to be particularly extreme.

Criticism of the DSM-5 (particularly from the American Psychological Association and the American Counseling Association) has focussed on the expansion of diagnostic criteria which may lead to an increase of mentally ill individuals and a pathologisation of normal behaviour with the result that ever larger number of people may be exposed to medications that can cause more harm than good. The DSM may also lead to treatment guidelines that recommend medication, and insurance companies may require diagnoses for medications in order to cover psychiatric services and also drug companies might aggressively market their products for these new indications.

It seems clear that a diagnostic manual will never capture the full spectrum of psychiatric disorders and, as Dutch psychiatrist Jim van Os argues, that psychiatry should be seen as a "complexity science" that embraces "not knowing". In an interview with the magazine *Vrij Nederland*, he is quoted in saying "If you are ready to think I don't know and we will explore together because the mind is complex you really help people" (February 5, 2024).

The problem with most medication is that the labels like "antipsychotics" and "antidepressants" are seriously misleading. The "antipsychotics" do not combat or cure "psychosis" and "antidepressants" do not combat or cure depression or "bipolar mood disorder". They are in fact neuroleptics – drugs that chemically control the nervous system. These psychiatric drugs are very powerful and addictive tranquilisers. They frequently make people look and act apathetic, zombie-like as if they've been lobotomised – even at moderate or low doses. These allegedly "safe and effective medications" always produce painful and serious side effects, some are health-threatening and brain-damaging; others are life-threatening.

Elaborating on this train of thought, we can refer to the much-discussed relationship between mental health and social stress. We are tightrope walkers; we need to maintain our balance ("homeostasis"). A threat to balance can be caused by multiple factors, physiological, psychological or environmental. In cases of acute stress – the attack of a lion – we have amazing mechanisms – stress receptors – to restore balance. In modern societies, you no longer have lions running after you – but there are chronic stressors, such as "will I be able to pay the rent at the end of the month?" We have great stress receptors, but, if the stress is chronic, it causes chronic inflammation, which in turn is a major cause of cardiovascular disease and mental disorders, such as depression. Several factors can cause depression, but the main player is chronic stress. And modern societies are organised to maintain constant stress levels.

Social chronic stressors include:

- Aggression and violence in our neighbourhood environment
- Income inequality and financial worries
- Differences in social status. Social inequality places us in a hierarchy in which we are ranked from good to bad. It creates the illusion that certain people at the top

are very important and certain people at the bottom are almost worthless. There-fore, in an unequal society, there is more status anxiety. This is a form of stress about what place you occupy on the social ladder, which in turn creates more bul-lying behaviour, insecurity, narcissism and so on.

- Competition in the work environment, distrust among colleagues and constant evaluations. Racial injustice, discrimination and exclusion

An interesting stress factor is also the pressure on consumers to make choices. Across soci-ety, we are faced with a bewildering array of products and services to choose from. The cost of living in times of endless options is anxiety and depression, because your choices can turn out to be disastrous. The paradox of choice culture is that it is at the heart of a consumerism that is part of a capitalist social order that does not offer a choice to reject it.

If mental health is not primarily an individual problem but a societal one, then the key question is: how can society adapt to our human needs? To this end, we should then learn in the face of competitive pressures the pleasure of non-competitive behaviour. Control choice stress by drastically curtailing consumerism. Replace increasing indi-vidualisation with more small-scale communal connections and train psychiatrists not as bio-technicians but as social activists.

Sane in an Insane Society?
The question Erich Fromm asks in his book *The Sane Society* is – can you be [mentally] healthy in a [mentally] unhealthy society? I think an answer to the question starts with thinking about what we can see as essential human needs and with an analysis of the relationships between human needs and human realities.

HUMAN NEEDS	HUMAN REALITIES
COMMUNITY	ISOLATION
CONNECTION	INDIVIDUALISM
LOVE	HATE
CREATIVITY	CONFORMITY

We could define mental health as the ability to belong, to love and to be creative. But the ability to meet these non-biological needs depends not only on the individual but also on how society is organised, which is how people relate to each other. Conclusion: to achieve mental health, social reality must adapt to our essential needs. As a result, mental health care should not be an adaptation to society but a social adaptation to human needs.

Within the neoliberal social order, mental disorder is seen primarily as an individual illness to be corrected rather than as a problem of the social order itself. Recently, admittedly, the idea of psychiatric illness has shifted from a strictly biological model to a biopsychosocial model that includes things like social conditions and life experience.

Workings of the Human Mind
Problems in mental health care go back to our limited understanding of how the mind works. The human mind is like a tropical rain forest in which everything is related to everything else (interdependence), where small events may have big and unpredictable effects (non-linearity) and where one cannot make reliable forecasts as flows of ideas

and opinion may unexpectedly and rapidly change (uncertainty). The human mind is a complex system. It is a collection (universe) of interacting agents that compete for a scarcity of essential resources (like space in traffic or oxygen and glucose in cancer cells). Characteristic of such systems is a mixture of order and disorder. Without a central controller, the emerging disorder (the traffic jam) may resolve as if nothing had happened and without external interference. The traffic jam appears for no reason and then disappears again, and this cannot be understood by deterministic or reductionistic thinking. Reductionism proposes that, by analysing and understanding parts of a system (as parts of a clock), we understand the whole system. However, this does not work with complex systems where we have to accept that a great part of our reality is fundamentally unpredictable. Determinism proposes that it is possible to establish linear causal relations between phenomena in our physical and non-physical environments. Causality assumes a simple world of one-to-one linear relations. More often than not, scientists can only demonstrate (with grave reservations) a correlation, an association and then speculate, hypothesise and guess. The "causality obsession" is fatal for a realistic understanding of the world in which we live. We live in a reality of multiple causalities, and it is probably impossible ever to single out one specific causal factor. The human brain does not follow simple cause-effect linear models. Reductionism and determinism offer an attractive simplicity that suggest we control the phenomena we investigate. This may be psychologically comforting, but it does not provide us with reliable knowledge. The acquisition of knowledge requires time. Understanding the human mind requires patience.

Human Rights-based Mental Health Care

As important features of a human rights based mental health care, the following could be listed.

Mental health and the failing realisation of fundamental social, economic and political rights. This renders mental health more than a health issue. It requires the management of modern societies in such ways as to enhance social conditions (like gainful employment) for people with mental vulnerabilities to enjoy the right to health.

Stigma and discrimination. There is a need to deal with the many misconceptions and the stereotypical images around mental health that have been largely responsible for creating and perpetuating stigma and discrimination. These include beliefs such as that mental health conditions are evidence of personal weakness or that having mental health conditions means that people are totally incapable of exercising agency over decisions that affect them and that they do not contribute positively to society.

Systematic training and awareness-raising for mental health personnel on human rights. This is needed to address the misconceptions that impede adequate mental health care. Training also needs to be directed at policymakers to combat the profound discrimination and inequality they experience. Such discrimination is now more widely acknowledged, among other discriminations in laws that prevent people with mental health issues from exercising human rights, such as the right to work and the right to vote

Informed consent. The right of patients to be involved in medical decisions should be guaranteed by providing complete information on the nature, consequences, benefits and risks of the treatment, on any harm associated with it and on the availability of alternatives. The guaranty of informed consent is a fundamental feature of respecting an individual's autonomy, self-determination and human dignity.

Many practices within mental health institutions contravene articles 15, 16 and 17 of the Convention on the Rights of Persons with Disabilities (CRPD). They include practices such as solitary confinement, forced sterilisation, the use of restraints, forced medication and overmedication.

The Right to Mental Health Among Vulnerable Populations

In this part of the chapter, we propose to analyse the right to mental health of vulnerable populations affected by armed conflicts, emergencies or disasters. In low- and middle-income countries (LMIC), mental health calls for action in the public agenda due to the worsening of psychosocial problems that affect life in society, such as the high indicators of gender violence, the increase in depression and suicide, the aftermath of armed conflicts and disasters, plus the havoc left by the COVID-19 pandemic. Concretely, in the current post-pandemic context, a high percentage of the population with mental health conditions have found themselves in conditions of greater poverty and inequality, having normalised living in exclusion, surviving on the edges. The challenge, therefore, is not only to generate decent living conditions and services for people with mental disorders but also to sensitise society in order to change behaviours, ideas and beliefs that promote situations of stigma, inequality, violence and social exclusion and thus contribute to the well-being and mental health of society as a whole.

Global advances in politics of mental health and human rights generate the illusion that more services are being offered to populations. However, reality show us that reforms in health services or law proposals are not enough, as core aspects such as human rights, respect, dignity and social inclusion (closely intertwined with mental health and well-being) continue to be affected by current conflicts and multiple systems of oppression. At the same time, living in unequal societies perpetuates a form of relationship in which there is always a group of the population that is kept in the margins outside of basic social services. Although the protection of mental health is the responsibility of states, there is little action. For instance, in Perú, one in five people experience mental health problems (Castillo-Martell & Cutipé-Cárdenas, 2019), and this is becoming more evident in people living in poverty and in victims of the internal armed conflict (Toyama et al., 2017). But, national states have stepped backwards in ensuring basic social services, reducing drastically their actions on behalf of victims of human rights abuses and the more vulnerable ones. Consequently, there's a need to advocate for approaching mental health as a human right. This means addressing people as subjects of rights and ensuring the protection of their mental health, contesting neoliberal and individualistic approaches that pretend to put the burden of the impact of social problems on the population itself, particularly when addressing persons who have gone through human rights abuses. Here, we reflect on the importance of rebuilding social and community ties that strengthen social networks and community belongingness in order to enhance local (individual and collective) capabilities (Rivera-Holguín & Velázquez, 2021).

In Latin-American countries we find many examples of how victims of human rights abuses are not being addressed as citizens and thus are not able to access basic social services or justice or redress. But, also, in Latin-American countries there are several experiences of resistance and collective organisation that aim to contest the trend of leaving behind the victims of human rights abuses, for instance, experiences that depict the diverse cultural understandings of mental health (what is mental health, how to seek for help, healing practices, cultural coping), the importance of the local collective organisations, and the core role that participation takes when referring to mental health.

Two Case Studies
The Sepur Zarco Case in Guatemala

At the beginning of 1982, in the Polochic Valley, the Sepur Zarco military base was responsible for the disappearance and death of a multitude of community leaders. The wives of these assassinated or disappeared leaders were forced to work in conditions of sexual and domestic slavery in the service of the military of the military base. Deprived of their freedom, they had to wash, iron, cook and do other domestic chores and were then sexually abused, first by the higher-ranked officers and then by the lower-ranked officers, in a systematic way, also being forced to ingest contraceptive pills and injections (Ríos & Brocate, 2017). The international legal sentence in this case was handed down on 26 February 2016 and included the classification of the sexual violence perpetrated as a crime against humanity. It is considered that the legal sentence expresses an important element that dialogues with a community model in that it demands that reparation be directed to the community as a whole and not only to the direct victims of sexual violence, ordering five actions that are oriented towards the recomposition of the social fabric and the reparation of the damage, which shows that the consequences of the human rights abuses impacted the community as a whole (Ríos & Brocate, 2017).

Case of the Santa Barbara Massacre in Peru

Santa Barbara is a high Andean rural community in Peru which, like many other communities, was affected by the internal armed conflict between 1980 and 2000. On 2 July 1991, two Peruvian army patrols arrived in Santa Barbara to raid a family; they accused them of supporting the Shining Path subversive movement. The family consisted of two elderly persons, four women (one of them pregnant), two men and seven children under 8 years old. They burnt their houses, stole their goods and animals, murdered people and blew up their bodies. The surviving family members have struggled for more than 20 years and in their search for justice have been accused of terrorism, imprisoned, tortured and threatened. All of them have suffered forms of physical and/or psychological torture in direct relation to the disappearance of their families. As described by the Truth and Reconciliation Commission (2003), most of the human rights violations in Peru were carried out against Indigenous Quechua-speakers. Despite this, most of the justice procedures and regulations do not take this diversity factor into account, which is why it is of particular interest to us to review the Inter American Human Rights Court's (IACHR) actions in this case. The International Court ruled on 21 November 2016, among other points, on the deficient actions of the Peruvian justice system in the investigation and lack of respect for the fundamental rights of the victims and their families, considering also the concealment of fundamental information by the Armed Forces and the excessive incompetence of the military jurisdiction to investigate the violation of human rights. In the same way, the delay of 24 years from the time the events occurred to the clarification of what happened and the search for the disappeared was considered a serious fault, thus concealing the truth from the relatives and the community, as an attempt was made to erase the evidence.

All these abuses had a serious impact on the mental health of the surviving family members and the community.

Concluding Remarks

Mental health includes the ability to enjoy physical, mental and social well-being; this definition moves beyond from the dichotomy between physical and mental health. Mental health includes a relational and a connectedness realm: feeling good about oneself and the people around you. Furthermore, mental health is related to the possibility to act in one's environment, to get involved in diverse initiatives and to find meaning in the things one is engaged in. Mental health problems cannot be reduced to mental disorders or clinical services, yet it also involves needs linked to psychosocial issues such as inequality, violence, poverty and corruption: domains that represent alarming situations and threats in the Global South.

Mental health requires a multilevel and psychosocial understanding that responds to the interdependence of human rights, which may benefit everyone in a sustainable way.

Mental health must go beyond treatment of clinical cases and integrate a perspective of prevention, promotion and care, that is, with a focus on mitigating and addressing long-term mental health problems (Rahman et al., 2021).

Mental health actions need to be based upon an understanding of the victims in their context and their daily stressors. Addressing mental health includes focusing on participation and agency of victims (Rivera-Holguín & Velázquez, 2021).

Mental health as a human right must move towards a victim-centred approach, where the relational understandings and empathy are underscored in order to contest the oppression and the degradation imposed by the human rights abuses. Focusing on dignifying relationships can contribute to repairing the damage of the social fabric, as well as the inclusion of victims' proposals and new methodological approaches (in which the holistic dimension of mental health is at the centre).

Human rights can inspire efforts to engage in forms of therapeutic relationships that are based on trust and empowerment. To this end, the links among psychiatry, public health and social sciences need to be strengthened so that new roles for psychiatry in shifting the profession from a controlling to a facilitative role can be explored. CRPD could be used to attain the highest standard of mental health care by strengthening the management and governance of health and social services. Psychiatrists and other mental health workers can play a crucial role in implementing human rights. A contribution from psychiatry was largely missing during the negotiation of the CRPD, but in its implementation psychiatry must be – and must be seen to be – a present and engaged partner.

Questions for Discussion

The objective is to reflect on and analyse the two cases from two angles: mental health impact and human rights. Please considering the following guiding questions:

- What do you think is the main cause of violence and why?
- How can we apply a human rights and victim-centred approach?
- What participatory strategies can you develop with affected people and their communities?

References

Abu-Raiya, H. (2015). Working with religious Muslim clients: A dynamic, Qura'nic-based model of psychotherapy. *Spirituality in Clinical Practice, 2*, 120–133.

Afolabi, A. B., & Joy, A. O. (2014). Confronting negative thoughts using Meseron therapy: A clinician approach. *IFE PsychologIA: An International Journal, 22*(2), 125–128.

Castillo-Martell, H., & Cutipé-Cárdenas, Y. (2019). Implementation, initial results, and sustainability of the mental health services reform in Peru, 2013–2018. *Revista Peruana de Medicina Experimental y Salud Pública, 36*(2), 326–333.

Fromm, E. (1956). *The sane society.* Routledge.

Ríos, J. & Brocate, R. (2017). Violencia Sexual Como Crimen de Lesa Humanidad: Los Casos de Guatemala y Perú/Sexual violence as a crime against humanity: The cases of Guatemala and Peru. *Revista CIDOB d'Afers Internacionals, 117*, 79–100.

Rivera-Holguín, M., & Velázquez, T. (2021). Las víctimas del conflicto armado interno y las reparaciones en salud mental. Propuestas desde lo comunitario. In I. Jave (Ed.), *La humillación y la urgencia. Políticas de reparación posconflicto en el Perú* (pp. 61–94). Instituto de Democracia y Derechos Humanos de la Pontificia Universidad Católica del Perú y Fondo Editorial Pontificia Universidad Católica del Perú.

Toyama, M., Castillo, H., Galea, J. T., Brandt, L. R., Mendoza, M., Herrera, V., Mitrani, M., Cutipé, Y., Cavero, V., Diez-Canseco, F., & Miranda, J. J. (2017). Peruvian mental health reform: A framework for scaling-up mental health services. *International Journal of Health Policy and Management, 6*(9), 501–508.

Van Dyk, G. A. J., & Nefale, M. (2005). The split-ego experience of Africans: Ubuntu therapy as a healing alternative. *Journal of Psychotherapy Integration, 15*, 48–66.

For Further Reading

Bolton, D. (2008). *What is mental disorder?* Oxford University Press.

Breggin, P. R., & Cohen, D. (1999). *Your drug may be your problem.* Perseus Books.

Burgess, R. (2024). *Rethinking global health frameworks of power.* Routledge.

Choudhry, F. R. (2016). Beliefs and perception about mental health issues: A meta-synthesis. *Neuropsychiatric Disease and Treatment, 12*, 2807–2818.

Council of Europe. (2000). *"White paper" on the protection of the human rights and dignity of people suffering from mental disorder, especially those placed as involuntary patients in a psychiatric establishment.* Council of Europe.

Lewis, O. (2013). The role of global psychiatry in advancing human rights. *Torture in Healthcare Settings: Reflections on the Special Rapporteur on Torture's*, 247–262.

Lewis, O., & Callard, F. (2017). The World Psychiatric Association's "bill of rights": A curious contribution to human rights. *International Journal of Mental Health, 46*(3), 157–167.

Rahman, M., Ahmed, R., Moitra, M., Damschroder, L., Brownson, R., Chorpita, B., Idele, P., Gohar, F., Huang, K. Y., Saxena, S., Lai, J., Peterson, S. S., Harper, G., McKay, M., Amugune, B., Esho, T., Ronen, K., Othieno, C., & Kumar, M. (2021). Mental distress and human rights violations during COVID-19: A rapid review of the evidence informing rights, mental health needs, and public policy around vulnerable populations. *Frontiers in Psychiatry, 11*, 603875.

Rivera-Holguín, M., & Velázquez, T. (2017). Bienestar emocional: Clave para la justicia comunal. In J. Ansión, A. Peña, M. Rivera-Holguín, & A. M. Villacorta (Eds.), *Justicia Intercultural y Bienestar Emocional: Reestableciendo vínculos* (pp. 161–192). Fondo Editorial PUCP.

Rivera-Holguín, M., Velázquez, T., & Otero, D. (2020). Aportes desde el modelo comunitario al abordaje de la tortura y la violencia política en Latinoamérica. In F. de Sa e Silva, P. Engstrom, & V. Hinestroza Arenas (Eds.), *Respondiendo a la tortura: Perspectivas latinoamericanas sobre un desafío global* (pp. 256–283). International Bar Association's Human Rights Institute, Universidad Externado.

Weitz, D. (2008). Struggling against psychiatry's human rights violations – an antipsychiatry perspective. *Radical Psychology, 7*, 1–9.

WHO. (2018). *Mental health, human rights and standards of care: Assessment of the quality of institutional care for adults with psychosocial and intellectual disabilities in the WHO European region.* World Health Organization.

WHO. (2021a). *Guidance on community mental health services: Promoting person-centred and rights-based approaches.* https://iris.who.int/handle/10665/341648

WHO. (2021b). *Mental health crisis services: Promoting person-centred and rights-based approaches.* https://iris.who.int/bitstream/handle/10665/341637/9789240025721-eng.pdf

WHO. (2022). *World mental health report: Transforming mental health for all.* http://hdl.handle.net/10713/20295

CHAPTER 8

Children and the Right to Health

Cees J. Hamelink and Victòria Fumadó

Introduction

On 20 November 1989, the UN General Assembly (in resolution 44/25) adopted unanimously the Convention on the Rights of the Child. With this convention, children became, in their own right, subjects of international law. Although there had been declarations on the rights of the child by the League of Nations already in 1924 and by the UN in 1959, it was felt by some UN member states that these rights should be brought under the authority of binding international law. The convention has been ratified by all UN member states with the exceptions of the USA and Somalia. The parties to the convention have accepted the obligation to undertake all appropriate legislative, administrative and other measures for the implementation of the rights recognised in the convention. The almost unanimous ratification of the Convention on the Rights of the Child by the international community does represent a major advance in the promotion and protection of standards to guide society's treatment of those under the age of 18.

Learning Objectives
After studying this chapter you will be able to:

- Understand the significance of the 1989 Convention on the Rights of the Child
- Analyse health problems that are specific to children
- Discuss parental, guardian and governmental obligation in relation to the right to health for children
- Make proposals for more adequate health policies concerning the right to health for children
- Describe how socio-economic health disparities and unequal opportunities during childhood might be related
- Describe the difference between equality and equal opportunities or equity for children
- Discuss how equal opportunities (in school and health) can be seen as children's human rights

DOI: 10.4324/9781003408765-11

The Factsheet

According to the WHO, under-5 mortality rate has decreased by 60% between 1990 and 2020, dropping from 93 deaths per 1,000 live births to 37 in 2020. Yet, this progress is not evenly distributed. These figures go up to 74 on average in sub-Saharan Africa, thereby lagging far behind SDG target 3.2.1, reduce under-5 mortality to at least as few as 25 per 1,000 live births in every country. The most common causes of under-5 mortality remain lower respiratory infections, diarrhoea, preterm birth complications and intrapartum-related events. Most of the under-5 deaths were preventable with low-cost interventions, for example, an estimated 21% of under-5 mortality is due to vaccine-preventable diseases (Perin et al., 2022). Yet, mortality rates for adolescents (and youth up to 25 years of age) declined only modestly over the same period (Masquelier et al., 2021). Also, the stark reductions in child mortality contrast with the slow progress in reducing the global non-fatal disease burden among children and adolescents; again the highest morbidity is observed in the less affluent parts of the globe. For children under 5 years, congenital anomalies, protein–energy malnutrition and diarrheal diseases were significant causes of morbidity. For older children and adolescents, childhood behavioural disorders, asthma, anxiety disorders and depressive disorders were major contributors to morbidity (Guthold, 2021). Notably, ill-health, in particular the first 1,000 days after conception, can result in physical and cognitive development problems and ill-health later.

The Intentions

Through the adoption of this convention, the legal obligations of international human rights law were extended to include children. In a strictly formal manner, one could argue that this inclusion was unnecessary. The essential characteristic of human rights is their inclusive nature. Nobody is excluded, and this would seem to suggest that children are among the subjects of human rights provisions. However logical this may seem to be, in daily realities (around the world) distinctions are made between adults and children. Political systems around the globe treat adults and children in different ways. Article 21 of the Universal Declaration of Human Rights provides that "Everyone has the right to take part in the government of his country, directly or through freely chosen representatives". Even democratic societies do not extend this basic citizen's right to those under the age 18. One can easily find robust arguments to rationally defend this differentiation between adults and children. Such arguments usually refer to "what is good for children". They often go back to the Greek philosopher Plato, who was strongly against the thought that children should engage in philosophical reflection. In Book VII of *The Republic*, Plato proposes a differentiation between the adult world and the world of children. Engaging children in philosophy would, in his opinion, be destructive both for children and for philosophy. Since he believes children are incapable of philosophical thought, their engagement in it would lead to indifference, and the future Republic would be crowded with people who could not discuss and who would not be interested in discussion. By the way, in Plato's thinking there also was no place in philosophy for women and slaves. The exclusion of children from philosophical practice was intended for their "good". In reality, however, it was those defending this position who actually wanted the best for themselves and their future polity. This reflects the very common desire that children should develop in accordance with the expectations that adults have. Adults want to shape children's world according to their desire to control and manipulate the world. In this line of thought, children should not ask too many questions and should accept things as they are. In most parts of the world, this has become the prevailing educational model! Fortunately, there are those who disagree. For Lipman (1988, p. 14), for example, children's philosophy is the basis of a democratic society: if children are not given the opportunity to weigh and discuss both ends and means and their interrelationship, they are likely to become cynical about everything except their own well-being, and adults will not be slow to condemn them as "mindless little relativists".

If one agrees with John Dewey (1888), that democracy is more than the rule of the many and represents primarily a way of living together whereby all voices matter, then the capacity for autonomous thinking and for asking questions is basic to a democratic society. Since philosophy is primarily the asking of questions, children should be encouraged to engage with philosophy since they can often ask questions on topics that are all too evident for adults. The convention opens up new avenues here, as it wants to facilitate children's participation in public communication. The convention's legal provisions combined with the new possibilities of advanced information and communication technologies suggest an immense creative potential for the future of democratic societies. Children can help adults to understand that intelligence is more that the ability to provide answers to questions and solutions to problems. This limited understanding is almost daily demonstrated in television's endless presentation of "quiz" programmes. Even science and technology are today often presented in the format of testing how much people know. Children's programmes could further the understanding that much more important than knowing answers to questions is asking the right questions. The convention makes the adult–child distinction problematic, since it provides children with a series of entitlements that are essential to democratic citizenship, such as the right to free speech and the right to freedom of association. The convention allows children to establish their own political association (with its own beliefs and ideas), but the association would be excluded from the formal political arena. Children's entitlements to fundamental rights pose new challenges to thinking about the public sphere. In the literature on the public sphere, one finds the conception of the public sphere as a single space where society's public discourse is located. Against this position, others like Nancy Fraser argue that, since most societies are characterised by deep inequalities, a single public sphere will always be controlled by the privileged groups in society. They propose to think in terms of a plurality of competing publics. In this conception, subordinated groups organise their own subaltern counter-publics (Fraser, 1993, p. 14). If the public sphere is seen as single entity, then children are certainly among the less-privileged participants. And, indeed, children play no role of significance in the public sphere of most (if not all) societies. Does this provide an argument for the multiplicity of public spheres so that children can organise their own public sphere as a location where they can express opinions, share experiences and develop protest actions? Would this, however, not lead towards the creation of separatist enclaves to whose interests overall society would be conveniently immune? It would seem that children need to have their subaltern public sphere but should also be able to interact with other sub-publics and eventually contribute to the overall direction of society. A further complication is that, in the case that children's rights would be conceived of as citizens' rights, many children would be excluded. If human rights are conceived of as citizens' rights, then the common implication is that human rights standards are valid for national citizens only. However, in most countries there are large numbers of people who, for different reasons, cannot claim citizenship, such as asylum seekers or illegal aliens. Among those non-citizens are children who, because of this status, are denied the fundamental entitlements that the children's rights convention promises to them. The recognition of children's rights gives extra urgency to the legal debate about the validity of human rights standards beyond the public sphere. Human rights are still primarily seen as legal mechanisms that protect and empower people in the public sphere. They provide a defence against acts of governments against individuals. It remains a bone of legal contention whether human rights provisions can equally be reinforced when they are violated by private parties in people's private spheres. Yet, when one thinks about provisions to protect children's physical and mental integrity, it would seem that such protection is particularly needed in the private sphere of family life. Exactly where children should confidently expect security and warmth, they often experience harm done to them by parents or other guardians

Good Versus Right

The awarding of fundamental rights means that a list of entitlements to forms of decent and humane treatment is provided. The complication is that the list contains rights that may in certain circumstances conflict with each other or that collide with other pressing interests, such as parental care and responsibility in the case of children's rights. International treaties do not provide keys for the solution of such conflicts and dilemmas. As a result – in actual daily practice – solutions will be sought in a casuistic way, and often they have to be provided by courts of law. Since such solutions would ideally reflect the interests of all stakeholders involved, the casuistic approach needs a discursive method through which those affected try to find a consensual judgement on a given situation. This discursive approach is only meaningful once the rights as enlisted in the children's convention are put into the frame of a broader normative theory. To this end, it deserves exploring whether such a theory may be found in the political philosophy of John Rawls. Whatever the shortcomings of the Rawlsian argument may be, it certainly provides a crucial argument for the prioritising of rights over conceptions of the common good. The essence of his argument is that "Each person possesses an inviolability founded on justice that even the welfare of society as a whole cannot override" (Rawls, 1973, p. 3). And he concludes that "justice denies that the loss of freedom for some is made right by a greater good shared by others" (Rawls, 1973, p. 4). There is a tendency among politicians to be guided by their visions of what constitutes the common good, and, equally, many parents and other guardians tend to have compelling ideas about what is good for children. This prioritising of good over right finds a fertile philosophical ground in post-modernist forms of normative relativism and in consequentialist approaches to ethical issues in which the ultimate "good" goal sanctions the means deployed. In all fairness, it cannot be ignored that there may be very sensible conceptions of the good in society, like the protection of children against pornographic or violent imagery. However, a Rawlsian normative theory would propose that right always has priority over good. This is particularly important with regard to children because of the understandable inclination of their guardians to propose that what they perceive as good for children's welfare takes precedence over children's rights. Often this really means that the parent's conception of the good for children equals the welfare of the parents. The welfare of parents and other guardians might indeed seem better served by children who do not say things they do not want to hear, who do not want access to information deemed inappropriate for them, who would not have to be listened to and whose privacy does not constitute a serious concern. However, to be able to see one's own welfare as parent or guardian as secondary to children's rights is the essential challenge of the effort to move children's rights beyond mere intentions.

Moving Beyond Intentions: The Obstacles

The lack of enforcement – the weakest component of the international human rights regime is the lack of a solid and effective mechanism for the implementation of its provisions. People should be able to seek effective remedy when their human rights are violated. Unfortunately, such remedy does not exist today on the global level. The European region has a fairly effective system of human rights adjudication through its Court of Human Rights. The existing global arrangements, however, such as the UN Human Rights Commission and the committees that monitor the various human rights treaties, do not constitute an independent world tribunal where complaints can be treated with supra-national jurisdiction. The UN World Conference on Human Rights in Vienna in 1993 declared that "the promotion and protection of all human rights is a legitimate concern of the international community" (UN, 1993, p.1). In reality, however, the majority of UN member states have little interest in interference with their human rights record. In current world politics, states still maintain a large measure of sovereignty in the treatment of their citizens. This implies, among other things, that the committee that examines the implementation of the Convention on the Rights of the Child does not have the authority to receive individual complaints. This lack of detailed jurisdictional scrutiny on the international level implies most likely that provisions on children's rights will not be subject to such examination on the national level either. Many countries have various enforcement arrangements that address legal situations in which children want to complain about maltreatment by their parents or when they are accused of criminal conduct. Such mechanisms (such as children's help telephone lines or children's law centres) do not presently exist on the international level. Most critical in terms of enforcement is the extension of the protection of rights to include horizontal relations. Fundamental rights are often violated between private actors, such as children and parents or children and private school boards. The communication rights of children are most often violated within the family. The enforcement within the private sphere is both most difficult and most needed. In order to achieve this extension of the application of fundamental rights, jurisdictional changes – but also a great deal of education for both parents and children – would be required. Next to these procedural issues there are also complex conceptual issues that may put obstacles in the way of implementing the convention's legal standards. Children as subjects of rights pose an especially difficult issue. There is already a good deal of divergent opinion about the interpretation and application of human rights standards for adults; the disagreements are even stronger when it comes to children. This is largely due to the different cultural settings within which human rights are to be implemented. There is a continuing international controversy about a Western, liberal bias in the prevailing conception of human rights and the need to recognise non-Western interpretations of rights. The widely diverging cultural conceptions of parental responsibility, for example, make worldwide consensus very difficult, if not impossible. Parental responsibility is across the world conceived in rather permissive versus more restrictive ways. A related problem arises because of different interpretations of Article 3 of the convention, which provides that "the best interests of the child shall be a primary consideration". The definitions of what the best interests of children are will vary greatly across cultural borders. An extra complication concerns the age of children. In different parts of the world, people have different conceptions about ages at which children come of age. The core concept in the human rights regime is "human autonomy". Ideally, we conceive of rights holders as autonomous individuals. What does this mean in the case of children? Children are initially dependent upon parents or other guardians, but as they grow up they become, to greater or lesser degrees, independent beings. In the process of their growth, individual autonomy begins to emerge. Yet, as with adult human beings, there remains throughout life a level of dependence upon others, and the intriguing complexity of the recognition of human rights is to find the balance between dependence and autonomy. With regard to children's rights, this implies that parents and other guardians have the responsibility to facilitate the process of children becoming autonomous subjects. This often seems a thankless task. The facilitators need to make themselves redundant while not distancing themselves totally from the children. Facilitating requires presence but with limited options to express one's views, since the views of the children take precedence. It requires a fundamental change from a more common commanding mode of communicating to a more difficult listening mode. There is (like in the case of mentally incapacitated people) the inevitable tension between the right to autonomous decision-making and the capacity to take autonomous decisions. Too often, however, the claim to autonomy is easily overridden by the dependency argument. It needs to be realised, though, that the priority of autonomy over dependence-induced heteronomy is a fundamental normative standard in international human rights instruments. It follows that, in case dependence is prioritised over autonomy, a basic human entitlement is violated. The defence of this violation will need very strong, substantial arguments. The rights that the international community grants children stem from the body of international law and specifically from the Convention on the Rights of the Child. However, identifying children's rights with the law may in several countries raises enormous obstacles, since children in impoverished environments tend to see the law more as a tool of oppression than as an instrument of protection. African kids may experience, for example, that the support they provide for their families by hawking and begging makes them, for purposes of law enforcement, criminals who perform illegal acts. For many children around the world, the law represents what you cannot do, not what you are entitled to do, even less what others (including law enforcement officials) are not allowed to do to you. The implementation of children's rights should, therefore, go beyond the application of legal rules. Children need to see their rights as their own constructions, as conditions of daily life that they identified themselves as necessary for a better life. A good illustration of this approach is the 12 rights that were proposed in 1994 by young street workers in Dakar and that meanwhile have become the common framework for action planning by working children in Africa. Most children in the world do not know they have fundamental rights. The child-friendly version of the convention that UNICEF Canada produced is not yet accessible to all the world's children, and children's rights are not yet common in school programmes around the world. At the time the international human rights regime emerged, the prime concern was to provide protection of the rights of individuals against states. There was little attention to individual duties, as the common notion was that states did not need to be protected against individuals through the imposition of civic responsibilities. Over the past decades it has become increasingly clear that human rights are not only violated by states but also by individual parties and that individual rights need to be protected against the conduct of other individuals. This made it imperative to recognise the duties of individuals vis-a-vis the rights of other individuals. The Universal Declaration of Human Rights provides the moral basis for such duties, particularly in Articles 29 and 30. Article 29.1 states "Everyone has duties to the community in which alone the free and full development of his personality is possible", and Article 30 imposes upon everyone the duty to refrain from "any activity or act aimed at the destruction of the rights and freedoms" set forth in the declaration. Since individuals have both rights and duties under international law, the question of children's responsibilities in relation to their communication rights has to be addressed. Now that children are subjects of international law, they are entitled to the protection of fundamental rights, but they also have the obligation to respect and protect the rights and freedoms of others. What does this mean for communication rights? One more general obstacle to the transformation of intentions into practices is the limited understanding about human rights violations. There is abundant evidence that the most universal feature of human rights is their universal violation. Incessantly, fundamental human entitlements are violently ignored by states, by corporations and by individuals alike. In order to make any progress at all in the protection and implementation of human rights, the forces, interests and motives behind their violation need to be better understood. Therefore, it is essential to investigate the reasons that underlie the violations of children's rights. Can they be found in culture- or class-bound conceptions of parental care and responsibility? Can a factor be the convenience of children's exploitation for commercial, military or sexual purposes? Does the underestimation of the intellectual and emotional capabilities of children provide an explanation? Do artificial distinctions between childhood and adulthood play a role?

Children's Right to Health
In relation to the right to health, the Convention on the Rights of the Child has the following provisions.

Article 24
1. States Parties recognize the right of the child to the enjoyment of the highest attainable standard of health and to facilities for the treatment of illness and rehabilitation of health. States Parties shall strive to ensure that no child is deprived of his or her right of access to such health care services.
2. States Parties shall pursue full implementation of this right and, in particular, shall take appropriate measures:
   (a) To diminish infant and child mortality;
   (b) To ensure the provision of necessary medical assistance and health care to all children with emphasis on the development of primary health care;
   (c) To combat disease and malnutrition, including within the framework of primary health care, through, inter alia, the application of readily available technology and through the provision of adequate nutritious foods and clean drinking-water, taking into consideration the dangers and risks of environmental pollution;
   (d) To ensure appropriate pre-natal and post-natal health care for mothers;

(e) To ensure that all segments of society, in particular parents and children, are informed, have access to education and are supported in the use of basic knowledge of child health and nutrition, the advantages of breastfeeding, hygiene and environmental sanitation and the prevention of accidents;

(f) To develop preventive health care, guidance for parents and family planning education and services.

3. States Parties shall take all effective and appropriate measures with a view to abolishing traditional practices prejudicial to the health of children.

4. States Parties undertake to promote and encourage international co-operation with a view to achieving progressively the full realisation of the right recognised in the present article. In this regard, particular account shall be taken of the needs of developing countries.

Article 23

1. States Parties recognize that a mentally or physically disabled child should enjoy a full and decent life, in conditions which ensure dignity, promote self-reliance and facilitate the child's active participation in the community.

2. States Parties recognize the right of the disabled child to special care and shall encourage and ensure the extension, subject to available resources, to the eligible child and those responsible for his or her care, of assistance for which application is made and which is appropriate to the child's condition and to the circumstances of the parents or others caring for the child.

3. Recognizing the special needs of a disabled child, assistance extended in accordance with paragraph 2 of the present article shall be provided free of charge, whenever possible, taking into account the financial resources of the parents or others caring for the child, and shall be designed to ensure that the disabled child has effective access to and receives education, training, health care services, rehabilitation services, preparation for employment and recreation opportunities in a manner conducive to the child's achieving the fullest possible social integration and individual development, including his or her cultural and spiritual development

4. States Parties shall promote, in the spirit of international cooperation, the exchange of appropriate information in the field of preventive health care and of medical, psychological and functional treatment of disabled children, including dissemination of and access to information concerning methods of rehabilitation, education and vocational services, with the aim of enabling States Parties to improve their capabilities and skills and to widen their experience in these areas. In this regard, particular account shall be taken of the needs of developing countries.

These articles have to be seen in the context of general provisions on children's rights as articulated in the following articles:

Article 6

1. States Parties recognize that every child has the inherent right to life.

2. States Parties shall ensure to the maximum extent possible the survival and development of the child.

Article 17

States Parties recognize the important function performed by the mass media and shall ensure that the child has access to information and material from a diversity of national and international sources, especially those aimed at the promotion of his or her social, spiritual and moral well-being and physical and mental health.

Article 19

1. States Parties shall take all appropriate legislative, administrative, social and educational measures to protect the child from all forms of physical or mental violence, injury or abuse, neglect or negligent treatment, maltreatment or exploitation, including sexual abuse, while in the care of parent(s), legal guardian(s) or any other person who has the care of the child.

Article 27

States Parties recognize the right of every child to a standard of living adequate for the child's physical, mental, spiritual, moral and social development.

Article 32

1. States Parties recognize the right of the child to be protected from economic exploitation and from performing any work that is likely to be hazardous or to interfere with the child's education, or to be harmful to the child's health or physical, mental, spiritual, moral or social development.

Article 34

States Parties undertake to protect the child from all forms of sexual exploitation and sexual abuse. For these purposes, States Parties shall in particular take all appropriate national, bilateral and multilateral measures to prevent:

(a) The inducement or coercion of a child to engage in any unlawful sexual activity;
(b) The exploitative use of children in prostitution or other unlawful sexual practices;
(c) The exploitative use of children in pornographic performances and materials.

Article 37

States Parties shall ensure that:

(a) No child shall be subjected to torture or other cruel, inhuman or degrading treatment or punishment. Neither capital punishment nor life imprisonment without possibility of release shall be imposed for offences committed by persons below eighteen years of age;

Article 38

1. States Parties undertake to respect and to ensure respect for rules of international humanitarian law applicable to them in armed conflicts which are relevant to the child

Article 39
States Parties shall take all appropriate measures to promote physical and psychological recovery and social reintegration of a child victim of: any form of neglect, exploitation, or abuse; torture or any other form of cruel, inhuman or degrading treatment or punishment; or armed conflicts. Such recovery and reintegration shall take place in an environment which fosters the health, self-respect and dignity of the child.

Case Studies

Case 1: Psychological Rehabilitation of a Sierra Leonean Child Soldier: A Case Study
Introduction: in the context of protracted armed conflicts, such as that which devastated Sierra Leone in the 1990s, children are often recruited as soldiers and subjected to traumatic experiences that profoundly affect their mental health and psychological well-being. This case study presents the psychological rehabilitation process of a child soldier from Sierra Leone, highlighting the challenges faced and the strategies used for his recovery.

Patient history: our patient's name is Shangko. He was 12 years old when he arrived at the compound in Laka.

Context: Shangko was recruited by the rebel group in Sierra Leone at the age of nine. During this time as a soldier, he witnessed and participated in acts of extreme violence, including murder, rape and torture; he also had to kill a member of his family under the threat of his own death by the leader of the rebel group. After 3 years of service, Shangko was rescued by peacekeepers and taken to a rehabilitation centre on Laka Beach. Shangko, along with other children, first underwent a health examination, where a skin infection was detected and was duly treated with antibiotics. At the centre there were rules, and the "military" discipline to which they were accustomed was used to approach the children and to be able to treat the trauma they experienced. But, upon arriving at the centre, Shangko did not obey the centre's rules and constantly showed his discontent; at the same time, he always boasted about what he had done during his time with the rebels. But there was one day when candy was distributed and, due to a mistake, it ran out; he looked around and started crying uncontrollably. From that moment on, Shangko lowered his defences and the specialists began therapy.

Case presentation: Shangko was referred to a team of mental health professionals for treatment due to symptoms of post-traumatic stress disorder (PTSD), depression and severe anxiety. He had recurring flashbacks of traumatic events, nightmares, insomnia, hypervigilance and avoidance of situations that reminded him of his time as a soldier. In addition, he showed difficulties regulating his emotions and establishing social relationships.

Treatment Plan
1. Initial assessment: a thorough assessment of Shangko's mental health was conducted to understand the nature and severity of his symptoms, as well as his specific rehabilitation needs.
2. Individual therapy: trauma-focused cognitive behavioural therapy (CBT) was implemented to help Shangko process his traumatic experiences, identify and modify dysfunctional thoughts and develop effective coping strategies.

3. Play therapy: play therapy techniques were incorporated to allow Shangko to safely express his emotions and explore his thoughts and feelings through symbolic play and creativity.
4. Community rehabilitation: Shangko's participation in community activities and reintegration programs was encouraged to strengthen his sense of belonging and connection with his social environment. The population near the rehabilitation center contributed by participating in carpentry and mechanics workshops and teaching the trade of fishing. Shangko was especially motivated to learn how to fish.

Results: after several months of intensive treatment, Shangko showed significant improvement in his PTSD, depression and anxiety symptoms. He experienced a decrease in flashbacks and nightmares, as well as an improvement in his ability to regulate his emotions and relate to others. Furthermore, he was able to gradually reintegrate into his community and begin to rebuild his life with the support of some family members and his new job as a fisherman – and the formation of a network of rehabilitation services – that continue to help him.

Case 2: "Rehabilitation of a Malnourished Refugee Child in Lesbos"
Introduction: the Chios refugee camp in Greece has witnessed a humanitarian crisis due to the constant flow of refugees fleeing conflict and persecution in their home countries. During the years 2015–2016, among the challenges faced by residents of these camps is malnutrition, especially among children. This case study presents the rehabilitation process of a refugee child suffering from severe malnutrition in the Chios camp and how his recovery was carried out.

Patient history:

Name: Ahmad

Age: 3 years

Context: Ahmad arrived at the Chios refugee camp with his family after fleeing the war in Syria. During his time in the camp, Ahmad experienced severe food shortages and poor living conditions, resulting in a state of severe malnutrition.

Case presentation: Ahmad was referred to the health center within the refugee camp after his mother noticed signs of malnutrition, such as weight loss, extreme weakness and abdominal bloating. Medical evaluation revealed that Ahmad was suffering from acute malnutrition and was at risk of serious complications if he did not receive immediate treatment.

Malnutrition, especially chronic malnutrition, ends up having disastrous manifestations for children. In addition to affecting their growth, resulting in short stature, it also affects the central nervous system, with less development and loss of neurons that affect cognitive functions and intellectual capacity.

Treatment Plan
1. Nutritional assessment: a comprehensive assessment of Ahmad's nutritional status was conducted to determine the degree of malnutrition and specific treatment needs.

2. Therapeutic feeding: a therapeutic feeding regimen consisting of highly nutritious foods and vitamin supplements was initiated to help restore Ahmad's weight and health safely and gradually.
3. Medical monitoring: Ahmad was closely monitored by a medical team to monitor his progress, monitor for any complications and adjust treatment as necessary.
4. Psychological support: emotional and psychological support was provided to both Ahmad and his family to help them cope with the trauma of the war and the difficult situation in the refugee camp.
5. Nutrition education: nutrition education was provided to Ahmad's family so that they could learn to provide a balanced and healthy diet for him even in conditions of limited resources.

Results: after several weeks of intensive treatment, Ahmad showed significant improvement in his nutritional status. He steadily gained weight, regained his energy and vitality, and his symptoms of malnutrition gradually decreased. Additionally, Ahmad's family received proper nutrition training and were able to maintain a healthy diet for him, even in the challenging environment of the refugee camp. At the same time Ahmed need psychomotor stimulation, otherwise will be very difficult to achieve normal development.

Concluding Remarks

Most of the thinking about children's rights comes from adults. Even child-friendly versions of relevant texts are often produced by adults. There is an enormous risk in all these well-intended efforts that adults shape the children's world to serve adult interests. The crucial challenge that the Convention on the Rights of the Child poses to adults is to listen to children, to consult them and to make them active partners in shaping humanity's common future.

Questions for Discussion
- Discuss the importance of comprehensively addressing the mental health needs of child soldiers, with a focus on individualised therapy, family support and community support and their important role in rehabilitation. Question: what positive impact can appropriate intervention have on the lives of children affected by armed conflict?
- Discuss the possibility of effective rehabilitation in the case of child malnutrition in refugee camps. Identify the human rights standards in providing health care in similar crisis settings.
- Discuss whether you think the Convention on the Rights of the Child would be different if people under 18 had been involved in its drafting process.

References

Dewey, J. (1888). *The ethics of democracy*. Andres & Company Publishers.
Fraser, N. (1993). Rethinking the public sphere: A contribution to the critique if actually existing democracy. In B. Robbins (Ed.), *The phantom public sphere*. University of Minnesota Press.

Guthold, R., Johansson, E. W., Mathers, C. D., & Ross, D. A. (2021). Global and regional levels and trends of child and adolescent morbidity from 2000 to 2016: An analysis of years lost due to disability (YLDs). *BMJ Global Health*, 6(3), e004996.

Lipman, M. (1988). *Philosophy goes to school*. Temple University Press.

Masquelier, B., Hug, L., Sharrow, D., You, D., Mathers, C., Gerland, P., & Alkema, L. (2021). Global, regional, and national mortality trends in youth aged 15–24 years between 1990 and 2019: A systematic analysis. *The Lancet Global Health*, 9(4), e409–e417.

Perin, J., Mulick, A., Yeung, D., Villavicencio, F., Lopez, G., Strong, K. L., Prieto-Merino, D., Cousens, S., Black, R. E., & Liu, L. (2022). Global, regional, and national causes of under-5 mortality in 2000–19: An updated systematic analysis with implications for the sustainable development goals. *The Lancet Child & Adolescent Health*, 6(2), 106–115.

Rawls, J. (1973). *A theory of justice*. Oxford University Press.

UN. (1993). *Vienna Declaration and Programme of Action*. Adopted by the World Conference on Human Rights on 25 June 1993. https://www.ohchr.org/en/instruments-mechanisms/instruments/vienna-declaration-and-programme-action

CHAPTER 9

Elderly People and the Right to Health

Cees J. Hamelink and Bert Keizer

Introduction

> Population ageing is a global issue that needs to be addressed from a human-rights based approach. Older persons should be able to enjoy their rights fully and under equal conditions, without suffering age discrimination nor being victims of abandonment, mistreatment or violence.
>
> *Santiago de Chile, October 2017, Report of the*
> *International Conference on Human Rights of Older*
> *Persons and Non-Discrimination*

The world population is ageing. Today, one in ten people is now 60 years of age of older. By 2025, there will be 1.1 billion elderly people worldwide. Yet, as we study the international legal instruments, we have to conclude that older people are mainly seen as in need of protection and not as rights holders. There are very few legal provisions on the rights of elderly people to work; to be part of the life of a community and to be entitled to freedom, dignity and autonomy. Today no separate binding international treaty exists to protect the rights of people who are elderly.

Learning Objectives
After studying this chapter you will be able to:

- Analyse the problems of ageing populations around the world
- Argue why it is important to approach elderly care from a human rights perspective
- Understand why care for the elderly is often not a policy priority in health care politics
- Explore your own position in discussion on the right to die in dignity
- Develop arguments for a UN Convention on the Rights of Elderly People

DOI: 10.4324/9781003408765-12

VIDEO: a talk between Cees J. Hamelink & Bert Keizer; http://www.kaltura.com/tiny/lowe5

The Factsheet

According to WHO statistics, by 2030, one in six people in the world will be aged 60 years or over. At this time, the share of the population aged 60 years and over will increase from 1 billion in 2020 to 1.4 billion. By 2050, the world's population of people aged 60 years and older will double (2.1 billion). The number of persons aged 80 years or older is expected to triple between 2020 and 2050 to reach 426 million. And,

> while this shift in distribution of a country's population towards older ages – known as population ageing – started in high-income countries (for example in Japan 30% of the population is already over 60 years old), it is now low- and middle-income countries that are experiencing the greatest change. By 2050, two-thirds of the world's population over 60 years will live in low- and middle-income countries.

Societies in East and Southeast Asia are among the most rapidly aging societies in the world. The number of older persons in Hong Kong, Macau, Singapore and Mainland China will increase by 243% from 2005 to 2050 compared with the world's average of 113%.

Of course, there is no standard archetype for older individuals. Some 75-year-olds possess physical and mental capabilities akin to those of 30-year-olds, while others may face significant declines in functionality at younger ages. Common conditions in older adults include hearing loss, cataracts and vision problems, back and neck pain, osteoarthritis, chronic obstructive pulmonary disease (COPD), diabetes, depression and dementia. As people age, they are more likely to experience multiple conditions simultaneously. For example, in 2050 it is estimated that there will be over 1.3 billion people with type 2 diabetes. Additionally, older age is marked by the onset of complex health states known as geriatric syndromes. These syndromes often result from multiple underlying factors and include frailty, urinary incontinence, falls, delirium and pressure ulcers. Addressing health issues of the elderly requires health systems that are adapted to deal with the broad array of (multi-)morbidity. Most notably, this requires health systems that provide continuous and patient-centred health care in combination with a holistic public health approach to accommodate this broad spectrum of experiences and requirements among older populations.

The UN Decade of Healthy Ageing (2021–2030) focusses on the reduction of health inequities and the improvement of the lives of older people, their families and communities through collective action in four areas:

> changing how we think, feel and act towards age and ageism; developing communities in ways that foster the abilities of older people; delivering person-centred integrated care and primary health services responsive to older people; and providing older people who need it with access to quality long-term care.
>
> *(WHO, 2022)*

Cultural Perceptions on Ageing

Our perceptions on ageing result from mixtures of biological and social factors. Perceptions may differ from longevity in blue zone environments (where people live to 100) to damaged lives in crime-ridden, densely populated urban centres. Education, ethnicity, gender and income create a diversity of experiences in ageing. A crucial variable is also the diversity of cultural environments people live in and the ways in which they form narratives about age. People's perspectives on aging reflect the diversity of their cultures. They view the ageing process through the cultural lenses their societies provide to them. There is still much research needed to understand how in different cultural settings people have internalised views on ageing.

As perspectives of the elderly influence their attitudes towards their physical and social states, we have to find ways to improve the quality of life in ageing by fostering positive perceptions of the ageing process and changing negative perspectives. One way of understanding how people internalise cultural values is through theories and empirical research on sense-making. Individuals in independent versus interdependent cultural environments make different sense of their lives. They figure out what different things are important for them and adopt different goals in their development throughout their lives. As Fung (2013) writes,

> the sense of limited future time motivates older people to prioritise goals that aim at deriving emotional meaning from life. . . . I argue that in older age when future time is perceived as more limited, and/or when mortality is made salient, one can derive emotional meaning from life through affirming and internalizing the values of one's culture.

The Right to Health and Ageing

Perhaps the most significant action by the UN regarding the status of elderly people under international law began in 1978 when the UN proposed a World Assembly on Aging. This World Assembly was held in 1982 in Vienna and was attended by 124 nations. The Assembly established, for the first time, the "right to age" as a human right. The Assembly produced a Report, including a 40-page declaration affirming that the fundamental and inalienable rights included in the Universal Declaration of Human Rights apply fully to elderly people, as the Preamble of its International Plan of Action on Aging begins: "the countries gathered in the World Assembly on Aging, (1) Do solemnly reaffirm their belief that the fundamental and inalienable rights enshrined in the Universal Declaration of Human Rights apply fully and undiminishedly to the aging".

The content of the Vienna International Plan of Action on Aging goes beyond a recognition of the equal rights of elderly people in such areas as health and nutrition, housing and environment, social welfare, income security and employment and education and includes "many useful and innovative recommendations to assist and protect the elderly, to enhance their sense of well-being, and to increase their productivity in society". Further, a central theme of the Vienna Conference was that the experience of aging "is a cross-cultural one in which similarities outweigh differences". Accordingly, a major goal of the Assembly "was to encourage nation-states to take the special needs of the elderly into account in all aspects of policy development and implementation and to facilitate participation by the aged in society to the greatest possible extent".

Among the major specific recommendations made in the Assembly's Plan of Action are the following:

- The segregation of the elderly is to be avoided. In particular, housing arrangements for the aged must "assist in securing their social integration".
- Home care for elderly persons with health problems must be made available whenever feasible. More drastic and isolative measures such as hospitalisation are to be avoided as much as possible. Health care alternatives must be developed that will enable the elderly to live as independently as possible.
- Steps should be taken to smooth the way for transition from a full working life to retirement.
- Government policies should reject stereotypical concepts concerning the capabilities and needs of the aged, especially the notion that advanced age equals incapacity.
- The recognition of aging as a shared human experience must be reaffirmed, as must be general awareness of the aging process.
- Recognition of the value of old age in its own right as a time for reflection must be increased.

Not only is the Vienna Plan not binding for States Parties, but also noticeably absent from the Plan is any obligation on the states to review and revise their own domestic laws to better protect the rights of elderly people within their borders.

In 2000, the much-awaited Hague Convention on the International Protection of Adults was adopted. The purpose of the Hague Convention is to avoid or resolve international legal disputes over the care and custody of people "suffering an incapacity or insufficiency of their personal faculties" and their property. This convention ensures that legal planning tools, such as advanced medical directives executed in one's home country, are legally valid and enforceable. Such directives are considered especially important today as more and more older people travel internationally. Additional international documents exist to protect the rights of elderly people in other contexts as well. For example, elderly people are mentioned specifically as one of the "other groups" in such treaties as the Convention on the Elimination of All Forms of Discrimination Against Women, which says that States Parties shall extend social security to elderly women on a non-discriminatory basis, "particularly in cases of retirement, unemployment, sickness, invalidity and old age".

There are provisions in the Universal Declaration of Human Rights that refer to old age. Article 25(1) states:

> everyone has the right to a standard of living adequate for the health and well-being of himself and of his family, including food, clothing, housing and medical care and necessary social services, and the right to security in the event of unemployment, sickness, disability, widowhood, old age or other lack of livelihood in circumstances beyond his control.

Also the International Covenant on Civil and Political and the International Covenant on Economic Social and Cultural Rights refer to rights that are of particular interest to elderly people worldwide. Similarly, other international treaties and documents as well as regional instruments refer to groups of people, which may include elderly people as well. However, none of these treaties have afforded elderly people comprehensive and binding human rights protection.

Proposals for an elderly specific treaty have circulated for decades, beginning with a draft resolution presented to the UN General Assembly by Argentina in 1948. In 1991, the UN General Assembly issued the UN Principles for Older People which are grouped around the principles of independence, participation, care, self-fulfilment and dignity. Even with such principles elderly people have fared far worse than other groups in terms of international law protection. Old people have been ignored by the international community and have encountered myriad physical and social obstacles that have deprived them of rights and dignity under international law. In discussing and applying the rights of older people, a clarification must be made. These are not new or different rights, and the protection of older people should not disconnected from everybody else's human rights. The leading question is how the universal rights that people enjoy can become equally effective in the context of older age and how we can fight against biases that exist in laws, policies and practices. Human rights offer the theoretical and normative language to achieve this objective. This is not about only today's older generation. It is a shared concern, since everyone will one day become old. It's about revisiting the universal principles of human rights and seeing in which ways they are failing older people.

Interview with Bert Keizer[1]

Since we wanted to introduce in this chapter the practical experience in health and ageing of a medical professional who worked many years in geriatric care, we conducted the following interview with Bert Keizer, geriatrician and philosopher.

CH = Cees J. Hamelink
BK = Bert Keizer

CH. Could a core problem with realizing the right to health for elderly people be that – certainly in the Global North – old age is seen as undesirable? Even old people often seem to dislike old people.

BK. Yes, I believe that the dislike of old age, the fear of old age, certainly means a hindrance when it comes to spending time, energy, and most of all lots of money, on the care for elderly people.

CH. As medical technology progresses and people get older and older: do essential choices become more moral issues than technical questions?

BK. So far we have managed to circumnavigate this horrible question. How? By being sober and honest about the technical possibilities when it comes to interfering in old bodies. Nobody thinks a heart transplant is a sensible option for a person who is ninety-plus years old. The chances of success are too lean. But when we enter into a dearth of medical assistance, are we then going to favour the young mother of two young children above the aged grandfather? During the COVID epidemic Dutch Intensive Care Physicians drew up a guideline to answer precisely this question. And yes, grandfather would not be admitted to the Intensive Care unit. I must emphasise that the directive is much more nuanced than this crude formulation.

CH. Is suffering no longer an acceptable reality? We do not want to suffer and want to live longer. But does living longer not often imply more illnesses and more suffering?

BK. Whether suffering is acceptable or not, there is no way of avoiding it. It is alas an unalienable aspect of being stuck in our type of body. You owe nature a death is the saying. And not just "a" death. It is you who will have to die. Prolonging life has brought us many extra years but also an extra long decline at the end. So yes, if you live longer you will be besieged by an increase of disease and suffering.

CH. People with dementia often say the worst is the people around them who see them only as patient. The well-intended family members want to care whereas support is more necessary. Would dementing people not rather need support to find how the days can still be spent meaningfully than patronising care that sees the patient as pathetic and unable to do anything anymore?

BK. One cannot generalise about dementia. Every stage of the disease is different. And to make it even more difficult: every dementia patient is different. Obviously in the first years when one is still reasonably capable of looking after oneself and moving independently outside the home, all one needs is supportive care. In the later stages the intensity of caring will grow and usually this happens quite naturally. In the very last stages of the disease one usually needs institutional care. I don't find this a particularly worrying problem. What does worry me, is that very often the caregiving husband, wife, daughter or son, realises far too late that the situation is severely damaging to themselves. The hardest thing for loved ones is to admit that a nursing home is really the only solution. They usually come too late to this realisation.

CH. There seems to be in the Netherlands an increasing demand for palliative sedation and more physicians are likely to grant the request for it. How to distinguish between palliative sedation and euthanasia? Is a second opinion in cases of palliative sedation to be recommended?

BK. Euthanasia is the administering or handing of a lethal dose of medication to a patient by a doctor at the patient's request. Palliative sedation is lowering the level of consciousness in a patient whose symptoms cannot be relieved in any other way. Euthanasia is only possible if a considerable number of conditions are fulfilled. It happens within a strictly regulated judicial context and the procedure must be reported to the authorities. In case of euthanasia a second opinion must be sought from a doctor who is in no way involved in the case.

Every doctor may refuse to perform euthanasia without stating his or her reason. Palliative sedation is not a measure which a doctor can refuse, because it is an emergency measure taken in circumstances where the patient is suffering horribly and there is no other way in which the suffering can be alleviated. There is no special place for a second opinion here.

Summing up the differences: euthanasia means a sudden death embedded in lots of important formal procedures. It is optional. Palliative sedation is not optional, the result is a much more gradual process usually ending in death.

CH. In choices related to sedation and euthanasia, or to treatment or no further treatment, often the "quality of life" issue arises. But who decides that quality?

BK. The quality of life can only be appraised by the patient in question. There will be a give and take around the issue in the form of a dialogue between doctor, nurses, patient and loved ones. In such an exchange I find that one usually reaches a consensus, bearing in mind that each person has his or her own way of coping with suffering.

CH. In the euthanasia practice a prime question is whether the suffering is "unbearable and hopeless"; but can your life or your death depend on a physician who finds your suffering is hopeless?

BK. I think the phrase used in the law is "unbearable and without any prospect of improvement or recovery". The second condition: "unimprovable" or "incurable" is more readily ascertained than the first: "unbearable". Medical knowledge usually offers pretty accurate evaluations of the prospect of improvement or recovery.

"Unbearable" however harbours a distinctly, if not hopelessly, subjective reaction to a grievous situation. Doctors are allowed to grant a request for euthanasia when they find the unbearable aspect understandable. This unfortunately implies a certain arbitrariness in the whole procedure. Some doctors are lenient, others are strict.

CH. Experiments in the social sciences have shown that people are often unclear about what they want and err about their preferences. Yet, are choices in the end-of-life phase not often based upon the assumption that people know what they want and know how to prioritise options?

BK. The haunting question in cases of euthanasia is sometimes: does she or he realise what is at stake here? Is he or she in full command of his or her mental powers? One way of resolving this question is by a systematic perusal of the answers to these questions:

1. The patient must understand the nature of the disease and what the possible treatments are.
2. The patient must understand in what way he or she is being affected by the disease and what the treatment options are in his or her case.
3. The patient must be capable of forming a rational judgment about possible alternatives and about the consequences once a decision has been reached.
4. The patient must be able to make a consistent choice.

Not all these conditions are always fulfilled. In cases of dementia (1) and (2) are often very doubtful. But one should be adamant about (3) and (4). These criteria are derived from an article about this topic by Appelbaum and Grisso in the *Nederlands Tijdschrift voor Geneeskunde*.

CH. In bio-ethical and medico-ethical discussions the concept of human dignity – often seen as the core principle of human rights – plays an essential role. The concept however lacks a solid rational justification. Can it really provide moral guidance in end-of-life questions?

BK. "Human dignity" is a vague concept. It is rarely used in discussions about euthanasia. However, one can translate the vague notion into a clearly noticeable aspect of a person's life. Being dependent on others when it comes to: getting out of bed – washing yourself – getting dressed – visiting the toilet, cleaning yourself afterwards – eating – drinking – getting back into bed. To be totally, or even partly, dependent on others for the performing of these simple ministrations is by the vast majority of people experienced as a source of terrible suffering. They tend to use the term "the loss of my human dignity" when landing in such a helpless state. The depth of this suffering is often underestimated by people who can walk and talk and drive and wash and use the tram and go out for a meal etc. etc.

CH.   We make life plans. Should we make death plans?

BK.   We should at least realise that one day we shall have to die. Thinking about this all the time makes your life miserable, maybe even unlivable. But never thinking about it is no solution either. Surely there is an in-between course in which we sometimes discuss our hopes and fears about how our lives will end with our loved ones, friends, relatives etc. So we can tell them what we think is an acceptable last act. Think about funeral arrangements, organ donation and who could be your representative when you can no longer look after your own interests. Talking about all this we might also learn something about how our spouses, children, grandchildren, friends and relatives think about their last chapter and if they expect us to support them in some way when they end up in medical hands.

Cultural Perceptions of Dying

A universal experience for all human beings is that they are born and will die. However, in most cultures talking about birth is easier than talking about death. Although we all share the certainty that we shall one day come face-to-face with death, most humans would rather not contemplate the idea of reaching the ultimate end of our sojourn on earth. Thus, the most common response to the thought of one's death – or the death of other loved ones – is fear. Humans and other animals have an instinctive drive for self-preservation. Humans, however, have evolved advanced and complex cognitive abilities that enable them to not only be self-aware but also to anticipate future outcomes. These sophisticated cognitive abilities make possible the awareness of the inevitability of death – and that it can occur at any time. Thus, the friction between the desire for self-preservation and the awareness that death is inevitable and unpredictable can induce feelings of anxiety and terror whenever situations arise that remind them of their mortality.

Around the world, death is differently defined and has different meanings. In some cultural traditions, such as Hinduism, there exists a vision of a circular pattern of life and death where a person is thought to die and is reborn – even multiple times – with a new identity. In the Christian view of death, dying happens only once, but the deceased continue life in a spiritual way and this may be either in hell or heaven. It may also be believed that the death and the living continue in co-existence, like among some Native American groups. However cultural traditions define death, they all have different beliefs about how people should die. Such different conceptions of dying have important significance for whether or not people fear death, how they prepare for it, what funeral practices they prefer and how they engage in mourning.

Cultures vary widely in the magnitude to which fear of dying is expressed. Some cultures appear to manage the idea of dying comparatively well, whereas in other cultures the aversion to the idea of dying is extremely strong. In most of the societies in the West, defying death is often expressed in terms of resistance, like the fight against cancer. Contrary to this, Eastern cultures may accept death and view it as a mere transition and propose that the most effective way to defeat death is to accept it as a primary fact of life.

Various studies have found different death anxiety scores between – for example – Australians (with largely Western cultural viewpoints) and Malaysians with Eastern cultural beliefs about death or between African-Americans and Caucasian Americans with the latter showing greater fear of dying than their older African American counterparts. It has been suggested that death anxiety may be higher in Caucasian American elderly because the majority of them are likely to die in hospitals, nursing homes, hospices or other institutions (Aiken, 1994). Thus, older Caucasians may fear dying in hospitals or nursing homes where they are very likely to be isolated from family members.

A theory – contested as it is – that may throw some light on factors that underlie cultural differences related to death anxiety is terror management theory (Solomon et al., 2004). The theory proposes that both humans and other animals have an instinctive drive for self-preservation. Humans, however, have evolved advanced and complex cognitive abilities that make possible the awareness of the inevitability of death – and that it can occur at any time. The desire for self-preservation and the awareness of inevitable death causes fear, feelings of anxiety and terror, and much human behaviour is inspired by coping with the deep anxiety (or terror) of dying. This can have the effect that people tend to do whatever it takes to ensure that they stay alive. Staying alive contributes to the continuity and socialisation of the species because people so driven are more likely to want to have children and to raise them according to their society's acceptable standards. However, the same death anxiety can become a destructive force and could even result in both physical and mental problems.

The Convention on the Rights of Persons with Disabilities and Ageing
Since 2008, the UN Convention on the Rights of Persons with Disabilities (CRPD) has been in force. The convention has been ratified by 177 member states of the UN. As Kanter (2009) writes;

> Perhaps most importantly to the development of a treaty on the rights of elderly people, however, is that fact that the Convention on the Rights of Persons with Disabilities, represents a new model which invokes the inclusion of human, civil, and political rights together with social, economic, and cultural rights. It also represents a dramatic paradigm shift from the medical or social welfare model of disability that focuses on diagnosis and inability to the human rights model that focuses on capability and inclusion and ways to prevent and remove the attitudinal and structural barriers that prevent people with disabilities, young and old, from becoming members of our communities.

Kanter continues,

> The new Convention gives elderly people, their allies and advocates a tool to require governments to accept certain formal obligations within the human rights rubric, and to hold such governments accountable through the enforcement and monitoring provisions of the Convention and its Optional Protocol. As such, the new Convention on the Rights of Persons with Disabilities provides a viable model for a new and separate binding convention on the rights of elderly people.

We take this proposal of Kanter to the questions for discussion and question how the model of the CRPD can be used to draft a convention of the rights of elderly people. What specific provisions should this convention have beyond existing human rights treaties. One could think of the need to build the capacity within educational institutions to meet the standards of healthy ageing provisions in the training of geriatric professionals or provisions on the prolongation of human life that too often results in a prolongation of unnecessary suffering. An important issue to be accommodated is also the discrimination that many people with dementia – and their families – face in getting the services or the support they need. A UN convention on the right to health and ageing would give robust attention to the abuse and discrimination of elderly people due to restrictions in physical, mental and sensory capacities.

Concluding Remarks

The ageing of the world population is well documented. Yet, the human rights of the elderly and especially the right to health are insufficiently protected and lack effective enforcement. The World Report on Ageing and Health (WHO, 2015) recommends profound changes in the way health policies for ageing populations are formulated and services are provided. More adequate policies should take into account that there is no "typical" older person. As the report suggests,

> the diversity in the capacities and health needs of older people is not random, but rooted in events throughout the life course that can often be modified, underscoring the importance of a life-course approach. Though most older people will eventually experience multiple health problems, older age does not imply dependence.

This may provide a solid base for developing for a robust defence of the right to health for the elderly.

Questions for Discussion
- Can the model of the UN CRPD can be used to draft a convention of the rights of elderly people? What specific provisions should this convention have beyond existing human rights treaties?
- Argue the case of assisted death of a patient with dementia who asked for euthanasia when they were still "compos mentis". Apply the human rights method of ethics.
- Identify in your own environment different conceptions of death and dying.
- Discuss how young people could prepare for ageing.
- Discuss how we should prepare for dying with dignity.

Note
1 Bert Keizer is a geriatrician and philosopher.

References

Aiken, L. R. (1994). *Dying, death, and bereavement* (3rd ed.). Allyn & Bacon.

Fung, H. H. (2013). Aging in culture. *The Gerontologist*, 53(3), 369–377.

Kanter, A. S. (2009). The United Nations convention on the rights of persons with disabilities and its implications for the rights of elderly people under international law. *Georgia State University Law Review*, 25(3).

Solomon, S., Greenberg, J. L., & Pyszczynski, T. A. (2004). Lethal consumption: Death-denying materialism. In T. Kasser & A. D. Kanner (Eds.), *Psychology and consumer culture: The struggle for a good life in a materialistic world* (pp. 127–146). American Psychological Association.

WHO. (2015). *World report on ageing and health*. World Health Organization.

WHO. (2022). *Ageing and health*. https://www.who.int/news-room/fact-sheets/detail/ageing-and-health

For Further Reading

Gutterman, A. S. (2022). *Human rights of older persons*. Older Persons' Rights Project.

Inter-American Commission on Human Rights. (2022). *Human rights of the elderly and national protection systems in the Americas*. OAS. https://www.oas.org/en/iachr/reports/pdfs/2023/PersonasMayores_EN.pdf

Megret, F. (2011). The human rights of older persons: A growing challenge. In *Human rights law review* (Vol. 11). Oxford University Press.

Von Hülsen-Esch, A. (Ed.). (2022). *Cultural perspectives on aging: A different approach to old age and aging*. De Gruyter.

Indigenous Peoples' Human Rights and Health

Monserrat Vásquez Ladron de Guevara and Pilar M. d'Alò

Introduction

"Indigenous Peoples" as a term encompasses diverse social groups who share unique ethnic, social and cultural characteristics deeply tied to ancestral connections and an intrinsic unity with their lands. Indigenous peoples typically have a non-dominant status within the national context, often facing oppression, marginalisation, discrimination and challenges to their land and resource rights. Estimations by the International Work Group for Indigenous Affairs (IWGIA) (2019) indicate a population ranging between 250 to 600 million spread across over 5,000 Indigenous communities, speaking over 4,000 languages, constituting approximately 5% of the global population, and they safeguard most (80%) of global biodiversity (Food and Agriculture Organization of the United Nations (FAO), 2017).

The unique ancestral tie Indigenous People have is with the territory where they live or where their ancestors used to live before forced colonial exploitations, displacements and in many cases genocide (Durie, 2004; Gocke, 2013; World Bank, 2020). In other words, Indigenous Peoples and the violence to which they are subjected are directly related to colonialism and its ongoing mechanisms and to the efforts to organise and develop according to Indigenous populations' own criteria (Cox, 2017; UN, 2006). The livelihood, health and knowledge system of Indigenous Peoples – which includes cultural, health and other practices of social organisation – has therefore been marred by the enduring consequences of white supremacy and colonialism (Durie, 2004; Gocke, 2013; World Bank, 2020). In other words, the health, well-being and health practices of Indigenous Peoples are inextricably linked to the systemic violence and violations of self-determination they endure due to (settler) colonialism. In 1948, the UDHR aimed to ensure equal social justice, freedom and dignity for all. Discussions about discrimination and violence against Indigenous Peoples within the UN intensified in the 1980s, culminating in the UN Declaration on the Rights of Indigenous Peoples in 2007, including their right to health. Within the Western educational system, the historical narratives surrounding Indigenous Peoples' experiences, particularly the atrocities

DOI: 10.4324/9781003408765-13

committed during European colonisation, have been erased or minimised. This omission perpetuates a collective lack of awareness, leaving many individuals uninformed about the profound impact of colonisation on Indigenous communities. It is imperative to reintegrate these historical truths into educational curricula to foster a more comprehensive and accurate understanding of the past.

This chapter aims to unveil an often-untold part of history essential for comprehending Indigenous Peoples' human rights. The chapter introduces a discussion on colonialism and settler colonialism from the perspective of Indigenous Peoples and addresses the history of international treaties, from the earlier colonial moments to contemporary UN resolutions. Drawing on existing studies and personal experiences, we delve into the discrimination and violence faced by Indigenous Peoples globally. The uniqueness of the Indigenous Peoples' case lies at the intersection of gender, sexuality, race, class, legal status, health and ability. In examining these issues, we underscore the urgency of acknowledging and rectifying historical injustices systematically overlooked. We will conclude with a summary of the unique elements in the codification of contemporary Indigenous Peoples' rights and their persistent breach by nation-states.

Learning Objectives

After studying this chapter you will be able to:

- Discuss the historical processes that lead to understanding Indigenous Peoples as a legal group in need of international juridical recognition, protection and support
- Understand the rights of Indigenous Peoples based on an operational definition of "Indigenous Peoples" in international law and an overview of the rights of Indigenous Peoples that have been recognised internationally
- Understand the key elements of Indigenous Peoples rights, including their right to health
- Understand the need for Indigenous Peoples' Rights as well as their enforcement and implementation and how this is an urgent yet insufficiently attended matter for both Indigenous and non-Indigenous populations worldwide

Historical Perspective on the Human Rights of Indigenous Peoples

The creation of a single definition of "Indigenous Peoples" has proven difficult given the wide variety in regions, countries, cultures, history and social conditions. The UN Food and Agriculture Organisation (FAO) considers Indigenous Peoples based on their historical occupation of a specific territory, their voluntary preservation of unique cultural traits, their self-identification and recognition by others as a distinct group and their experiences of marginalisation or discrimination (FAO, n.d.)

There are two important elements to keep in mind when looking at the rights of Indigenous Peoples, also in relation to health: their long history but late, unique codification and the generalised lack of implementation, amid a few exceptional cases of good practice. This section is concerned with the first element, namely the historical process and key moments that led to the current definition and status of Indigenous Peoples' rights and the qualities that render them a one-of-a-kind type of human rights.

In the West, the journey to recognise and address the human rights of Indigenous Peoples traces back to post-World War II and the rapid independence of former colonies in Africa and Asia. Indigenous Peoples' activists, since the 1940s, began highlighting their systemic precarity and its ties to ongoing colonial processes. Despite their richness in resources and specific environmental knowledge, Indigenous ecosystems face fragility due to climate change, extractivism and urbanisation. The lands have been seized by state and private actors for meeting global demands for natural resources or to continue "green capitalism development" projects (Shelton, 2020). Activities like mining, oil drilling, forestry, energy transition projects, agriculture, livestock and water usage persistently contribute to forced displacement, assimilation, conflict and even continue genocide against Indigenous Peoples, all to satisfy global energy, "development", manufacturing and food needs or the comfortable living standards of the Global North.

Settler Colonialism from the Perspective of Indigenous Peoples

"Indigenous Peoples" is a key legal concept that has been increasingly codified by international law. As explained earlier, its conceptualisation emphasises the connection with the land and their continued dispossession due to continued processes of colonialism. Rodney (2018) provides a useful understanding of colonialism as a country's policy of extending and maintaining its political, economic, social and cultural authority over people and territories not part of the nation's initial organisations.

In this sense, colonialism is not a past event that took place and ended but is rather *an ongoing process* where the coloniser country continues to benefit from the colonised people and their lands' resources. At times, colonialism takes the shape of settler colonial societies. This is the case, theorised by Veracini (2010, 2013), where settlers from the coloniser state "constitute an autonomous political body" that substitutes the sovereignty of Indigenous social and political organisation (2010, p. 1).

Both colonialism and settler colonialism enforce dominance over the territories they colonised on and populations that lived there through a variety of violent methods with the effect of benefitting from the colonised labour and resources. However, Veracini marks an important distinction between these two forms of colonialism, insofar as the second specifically requires the intentional final disappearance of Indigenous people as they are progressively replaced by the settlers (Veracini, 2010).

Colonialism as a modern and yet uninterrupted continued system of dominance is considered to have started with the European expansion in the African and American territories during the 15th and 16th centuries. The colonial movement later also included the land east of Europe;[1] but the political, economic and epistemic shift that European powers experienced with 1492 is considered by many scholars the beginning of colonialism as the most defining experience of Modernity (Quijano, 2000). The European economy did not evolve spontaneously into capitalism and its racialised exclusions (Veracini, 2010). Rather, thanks to the categorisation of certain peoples, notably enslaved Africans and the Indigenous communities of the Americas, as less human than the (white) European colonising powers (Wynter, 2003), it was possible to justify enslaved labour and resource extraction.

What we want to highlight is that the expansion to the Americas, combined with the enslavement of African populations, meant the establishment of system of dominance and exploitation oriented towards the uneven circulation of wealth. This circuit was organised to benefit European ruling elites, leading to the transformation of economic dynamics and eventually to the development of modern nation-states and economic relations (Wynter, 2003; Rodney, 2018).

Militarisation, conflict, expulsion from lands due to commercial purposes and climate change, together with disproportionate poverty rates and inequality in access to health, housing, education, employment and land disposition (due to settler occupation and disposal), force Indigenous Peoples into moving and migration (Expert Mechanism on the Rights of Indigenous Peoples (EMRIP), 2019). The Expert Mechanism on the Rights of Indigenous Peoples points out how one of the main challenges related to migration is the territorial and cultural uprooting, which leads to even more vulnerability.

Moreover, insecure land tenure is a catalyst for conflicts, environmental degradation and socio-economic impoverishment (EMRIP, 2019). Social marginalisation both perpetrates and reproduces the forced displacement – and sometimes resettlement – of Indigenous populations (EMRIP, 2019). The Inter-American Commission on Human Rights (IACHR) in effect found (2000) that no other group has been hurt as much by historical violence as Indigenous Peoples. This is largely due to the general lack of formal recognition of ownership over their ancestral lands, territories and resources. Even when recognition is granted, state protection from external parties tends to be weak, if non-existent: Indigenous groups asserting their rights has often resulted in torture, imprisonment or death (UN Department of Economic and Social Affairs (UN DESA), 2012). EMRIP (2019) asserts that many of the issues Indigenous Peoples face – and many of the consequences their forced displacement and assimilation into dominant culture carry – are caused by the lack of recognition of Indigenous Peoples as independent subjects of international law and rights.

Finally, the different ways Indigenous Peoples have historically and geographically defined themselves complicates the design of targeted policies, laws or treaties. This stark reality emphasises the imperative for a legal framework that not only recognises Indigenous Peoples' historical dynamics but also empowers them through self-determination, offering a path towards addressing the root causes of their challenges and fostering a more just and equitable future. The issue of establishing a legal category is therefore crucial to Indigenous Peoples' survival, protection and condition bettering.

Early Colonial Treaties

The Americas is a region rich with early history of Indigenous Peoples' rights, insofar as it was the encounter with this region's populations that prompted European scholars to craft new legal criteria to define legitimate enslavement, serfdom, conquest, occupation or administration of people and territories. For the philosopher Sylvia Wynter, the encounter with the Americas was the moment that prompted European intellectual elites to re-define what humankind was altogether. Legal categories reflect those new definitions of what it meant to be human – and who met the standard. Moreover, they illustrate the relationship between those who were to be considered "human" and those who were categorised as "sub-human".[2] The first efforts by legal scholars to regulate the appropriate relationship between colonised and colonisers started to be debated as early as the 15th century, during the conquest of what became the American continent. At this time, European monarchies developed the legal categories of "rationality" and "irrationality" to determine if an Indigenous group was to be recognised as a sovereign entity (like European monarchies considered themselves) with whom to negotiate. To be a rational subject was to be able to make use of rationality and rise above impulses so to be properly able to govern oneself and others. To be recognised as "rational", as it happened for peoples in the Americas, meant to retain forms of sovereignty, and European law at the time forbid enslavement or direct conquest and submission.

Initially, particularly in the Americas,[3] Indigenous Peoples retained sovereignty over parts of their territory and negotiated land rights, trade, warfare and external relations through treaties (Shelton, 2020). First peoples were therefore granted formal ownership of their lands. However, in practice, even when legal scholars categorised the colonised as "rational beings", their status was most often considered that of children, not fit to the standard (see de Vitoria, 1917, p. 160 in Shelton, 2020, p. 218). Spain was therefore allowed to lawfully administer or conquer more territory. In the cases where the "rationality" of original populations was not recognised, as was often the case of African peoples, slavery and conquest of territory were fully justified by the European international law (Wynter, 2003). This is because standing outside the category of "rationality" meant to be associated with non-human animals rather than with children that could be educated.[4]

Crucially, these were legal categories that legitimated European powers to rule over others. The limitations to the exercise of sovereignty through the framework of "not completely rational" (in the Americas case) and completely "non-rational" in most African cases informs contemporary approaches to Indigenous People's rights. On the other hand, despite the racial and colonial classification, these initial relations represent a recognition of clearly demarcated Indigenous communities as sovereign entities that could participate with European powers in international law (Shelton, 2020). It is some of these early treaties and forms of recognition that, despite their systematic violation and racist formulation,[5] continue to form the basis of contemporary IP claims for collective land ownership and self-determination.

The 1900s Codifications in Law

In the 1920s at the League of Nations and after World War II with the establishment of the UN, a renewed focus on decolonisation and Indigenous populations emerged (Anaya, 2009; Singel, 2008). Indigenous Peoples were not yet discussed as a particular group or category deserving a specific codification. The League of nations recognised some rights of ethnic, religious and linguistic minorities, but Indigenous Peoples were generally excluded (Shelton, 2020).

Some progress was made in the Americas, where Indigenous Peoples were identified as an "issue" to be addressed (ibidem). Despite some regional advancements, the UN did not create a specific category of protection for Indigenous Peoples. Instead, Shelton (2020) reports how international legislation promoted formal decolonisation of the territories occupied by European powers in Africa and Asia, so the right to self-determination was only recognised for external territories and excluded groups inhabiting settler states (such as the US or other Latin American countries).

The 1957 International Labour Organisation (ILO) Convention No. 107 was the first international tool completely dedicated to the issue of Indigenous Peoples. The Convention configures the protection of individual rights and frames the problems faced by Indigenous Peoples as exploitation (Anaya, 2004). The framework was presented mostly as a matter of failed integration, indicating that often violent forms of assimilation were still not considered part of the problem. Swepston (2015) argues that ILO's Convention remained at the core an "assimilationist instrument aimed at ameliorating the most abusive practices by colonial powers" (Shelton, 2020, p. 220).

In 1989, the Indigenous and Tribal Peoples ILO Convention No. 169 reframed Indigenous Peoples' rights as rights of a community. Convention No. 169 focused on protecting and defending Indigenous Peoples by improving their living conditions via employment, health, education and land rights. Crucially, it did so by determining cultural and identity presentation in collective terms. While individual rights are rights held by each person individually even when differentiated by group, as it happens with gender-specific or ethnicity-related rights (Jones, 2016), collective rights are held by a group per se.

With a focus towards self-determination, identity and heritage, James Anaya finds the genealogical tie to "inhabitants of lands now dominated by others" (2004, p. 3) a determinant quality of "Indigenous" people, whereas "peoples" refers to "communities with an identity that connects them with their past ancestors (Ibidem)". In efforts to participate in their own recognition, many Indigenous Peoples themselves have placed the definition of their Indigeneity neither in colonisation nor in its legacy of impoverishment. Rather, it has been found in the deep feeling of connection with the environment and their long-term relationship with it (Durie, 2004).

As a result, Convention No. 169 (1989) and the 2005 World Bank Operational Directive 4.10 avoid the definition to focus on who is going to be covered by the convention (MacKay, 2005; Errico, 2006). In the World Bank document specifically, Indigenous Peoples is used in a generic way referring to distinct, vulnerable social and cultural groups that, to varying degrees, possess the following qualities: self-identification as members of an Indigenous group and recognition by others; collective tie to specific territories and to the natural resources of these territories; distinct cultural, economic, social and/or political institutions that differ from the dominant ones; a language that might be different from the official one(s) in the country or region (MacKay, 2005).

Contemporary Indigenous Peoples' Rights and Intercultural Care Practices

The 2007 UN Declaration on the Rights of Indigenous Peoples (UNDRIP) puts further emphasis on protecting Indigenous People in their communal identity and heritage. The Declaration establishes a framework of minimal standards required for survival, dignity and well-being of Indigenous Peoples. Addressing one of the most crucial aspects in Indigenous Peoples' rights, the Declaration remarks on the recognition of rights of peoples to be distinct, consider themselves as such, and be respected in that and frames this diversity as "richness" and "common heritage of humankind" (UN, 2007, pp. 2–4). Therefore, the fundamental importance of peoples' self-determination is highlighted, opening the route for them to "freely determine their political status and freely pursue their economic, social and cultural development" (Ibid., 6).

The 2007 Declaration covers these critical points for the protection and enforcement of Indigenous Peoples' rights by addressing state-Indigenous Peoples' relationships and state actions towards Indigenous Peoples. Aiming at creating cooperative relations between states and Indigenous Peoples, the 10 Declaration points directly to how states should interact with the document, namely indicating working together with the Indigenous communities for granting or improving their protection and self-determined development.

The relevance of repeatedly stressing concrete state action is not to be taken for granted. Indeed, one of the main obstacles to the development of the Declaration – and later to its adoption by the General Assembly – was precisely the kind of self-determination rights over lands and resources, when not political and economic, that the Declaration implied. The document declares any form of discrimination a violation of Indigenous Peoples' rights and promotes their effective participation in all matters concerning them. Finally, it is crucial to note that, while the Declaration has been signed by almost all UN State members, it remains non-legally binding.

Together with asserting the collective rights of Indigenous Peoples and indicating a solid path for state action, the Declaration addresses the following themes:

- Rights of self-determination as Indigenous individuals and as Indigenous Peoples (Articles 1–8; 33–34)
- Cultural rights and identity: the rights of Indigenous Peoples and individuals to determine, defend and engage in their cultural practices, languages, education and religion (Articles 9–16; 25, 31)
- Political rights: the rights to define, defend and engage in their own form of political and economic organisation (Articles 17–21; 35–37)
- Health rights (Articles 23–24): access to all the social and health services of the region and country where they reside, as well as the right to maintain their traditional medicine, since they have the right to attain all the highest standards of physical and mental health
- Labour rights (Articles 17, 21)
- Land rights: this includes issues such as ownership (i.e. reparation or return of land, Art. 10 among others) and environmental protection (Articles 26–30, 32)
- Protection of in-group vulnerable such as the elderly, women, children (Article 22)

It also indicates some concrete measures states should take so as to uphold the rights of Indigenous individuals and peoples:

- To return land (Article 26), ceremonial objects (Article 12) and human remains (Article 12)
- To place "programs for monitoring, maintaining, and restoring the health of Indigenous Peoples" (Article 29) both as a collective and as individuals

To assist UN Member States in achieving the UN Declaration goals, in 2007 (res. 6/36) the Expert Mechanism on the Rights of Indigenous Peoples was established as a subsidiary body of the Human Rights Council. The EMRIP's role is to conduct research to advance the protection and promotion of Indigenous Peoples' rights. It provides the Human Rights Council with expertise and advice on the rights of Indigenous Peoples, mostly by assisting the Member States in achieving the goals of the UNDRIP. It clarifies the implications of the main principles such as informed consent and self-determination; it examines good practices and challenges regarding the implementation of Indigenous Peoples' rights and it suggests laws, programs and policies to states and other responsible institutions.

A significant step forward for Indigenous rights in the Americas was adopted in 2016 when the IACHR adopted the American Declaration on the Rights of Indigenous

Peoples. The IACHR was particularly celebrated insofar as in the region Indigenous Peoples are highly active in defending their rights, communities, lands and resources from governments and (quite often) foreign extractive companies despite actual violence or threat of it (IACHR, 2017). Moreover, the legal practice in the Americas impacted international codification by giving "prominence to the collective and individual rights of indigenous peoples" (Shelton, 2020, p. 222).

The concepts of self-determination and property are defined in religious, cultural and economic terms as collective or group rights stemming from a history of marginalisation. Two basic tenets of human rights – individual enjoyment of civil, political, economic, social and cultural rights and that in specific social settings specific groups might require protection for their continued existence – served to reshape individual rights in the light of the specific challenges faced by Indigenous Peoples (ibid.: 222–4). In other words, the history of continued colonisation informs the codification into international law and jurisprudence of the subject of rights "Indigenous Peoples" as holders of very specific rights unique only to those human groups who can be classified as Indigenous Peoples. To treat Indigenous Peoples equally accordingly to international law is not just to recognise them as subjects of individual rights but requires the unique recognition of their distinctive collective culture, knowledge and forms of land property.

The progressive crafting of Indigenous Peoples' rights as a unique type of *collective* right that is to be granted to a distinctive group goes hand in hand with state recognition of these groups and enforcement of their rights. This implied for settler coloniser states to give formal acknowledgement and effective implementation of policies attending to Indigenous Peoples' historical marginalisation. The exceptionalism of Indigenous Peoples' human rights, Shelton calls it, implies a "reparative aspect" as direct response to colonial injustices, resulting from the effort of advocates and Indigenous leaders in their interaction with Inter-American Courts (2020, p. 226).

Indigenous Peoples' Self-determination: Land, Culture and Collective Personhood

Indigenous Peoples' self-determination encompasses vital aspects such as land, culture and collective personhood. Before discussing the inadequate responses of states and their subpar practices, it's essential to highlight the distinctive qualities of Indigenous Peoples' rights. According to Shelton (2020), the right to property has traditionally been conceptualised as an individual right. However, both IACHR and the Court have recognised this right in a manner that embraces a unique understanding of *collective* ownership of territory and utilisation of resources (225). This distinction arises from the historical use of land displacement and resource appropriation as mechanisms for imposing assimilation and perpetuating generational socio-economic impoverishment. Furthermore, the significance of territories and ecosystems extends beyond mere geography; they profoundly shape the entire socio-cultural and politico-economic organisation of Indigenous Peoples.

The relationship with nature and the natural world, which of course inform Indigenous Peoples' plea for land rights and ownership, is at the core of most Indigenous cosmologies, governance and knowledge systems, including education, health and wellbeing (Malezer, 2005; Loncon, 2023). It emerges quite clearly, as Indigenous thinkers have expressed (Durie, 2004), that Indigenous knowledge systems are based upon the environment where communities lived or live, including medicinal practices, agricultural techniques, food systems, biodiversity preservation, cultural production, cosmovision and political and social structures. The Inter-American Development Bank has reaffirmed that specific lands, environments and ecosystems define the *natural and social* space needed for the survival of Indigenous communities, both in physical and cultural terms (1997, p. 9).

We see here the interconnection among self-determination, cultural rights and land rights for the equality and non-discrimination of Indigenous Peoples. As Shelton argues (2020): "perhaps the most significant legal consequence flowing from acknowledgement of indigenous collective identity is the right to be recognised collectively as legal persons" (p. 227). Existing law and jurisprudence have qualified self-definition as fundamental to identifying Indigenous communities as holders of collective rights as well as forbidding assimilation. In other words, the right to self-determination guarantees a territorial integrity within the settler coloniser state and a degree of independent decision-making regarding such territory. It was the land to be invaded, and it is the land that offers cultural and economic well-being and structures a knowledge system and sense of identity. For this reason, land is pleaded as a right to *collective* ownership, not individual to single members of the group. And it follows that collective land ownership becomes the key legal, political, social, economic mechanism through which self-determination translates into effective practice.

However, the introduction of industrial agricultural technologies (i.e. chemicals as pesticides and fertilisers or large plantation schemes) or "development projects" (e.g., dam or pipeline construction) have demolished – when not erased – ecosystems that Indigenous communities had depended on, therefore forcing migration and resettlement (UN-DESA, 2009). Generally, governments have granted access to land and resources for extractive projects without Indigenous communities' informed consultation and consent or compensation.

More recently, within the global trends for ecological conservation, we see how Indigenous Peoples have been forced off their ancestral lands, also because of ecotourism and national park development (Ibid). This despite Indigenous communities' knowledge and practices recognition of their contribution to ecological integrity, biodiversity preservation and environmental health (Ibid.; FAO, 2017).

At the national level, public policies and laws need to address the mechanisms that reproduce Indigenous Peoples' state of systematic marginalisation to create structures where retribution is accompanied with the consciousness of past and present processes. Access to clean water, sanitation, housing, health, education, employment, land and resources must be guaranteed to any other human or citizen of a nation. Basic service access, moreover, needs to be accompanied by public investments in intercultural or culturally appropriate services (Rivera-Cusicanqui, 2010).

In conclusion, it is crucial to emphasise once more how the enterprise of colonialism and its enduring effects played a pivotal role in shaping the development of human rights. This perspective serves as a potent challenge to prevailing state practices, directly linked to exploitative colonial processes, the uneven distribution of resources and racial standards dictating notions of civilisation, humanness and development. Moreover, it prompts focus on how the formal recognition of rights remains contingent on the very states that exercise control over Indigenous Peoples and their territories. While innovative, Indigenous Peoples' rights have often been implemented differentially and frequently wielded to advance the agendas of former colonising countries (Samson, 2020). Their belated and incomplete acknowledgement still depends on the persisting colonial legacies of state formation, state policies, racial narratives of nationhood and the relentless pursuit of energetic and economic needs (Rivera-Cusicanqui, 2010). A critical examination of human rights unveils the non-universal history of their implementation, intricately tied to colonial interests.

Indigenous Peoples' Health and Intercultural Care Practices

It could be argued that one of the most striking indicators of Indigenous Peoples' systemic marginalisation and dispossession is their health status. Although the WHO points to the shortage of statistical data on the health of Indigenous Peoples (2007), when comparing country-specific research, a global trend emerges. In both Global North and Global South countries, Indigenous Peoples suffer worse health status than non-Indigenous populations in almost every health-related issue. In a study encompassing the US, Canada, Australia and New Zealand (Ring & Brown, 2003), for example, the health gap between Indigenous and non-Indigenous populations is evident, particularly for chronic diseases and related deaths, which account for over the 70% of mortality excess. The condition relates to the lack of access to primary, secondary and tertiary services, which implies that many health conditions are underdiagnosed and undertreated (Ibidem). To cite other instances, in Cambodia, 20% of Indigenous children under 5 years old suffer from malnutrition, and over 52% are stunted in growth (AIPP & UN-DESA, 2015). In Central Africa, where commercial poaching depletes natural resources, Pygmy communities are denied access to the land to grow food. They are currently facing food and nutrition insecurity (Ohenjo et al., 2006).

Worldwide, child mortality is higher for Indigenous populations than for non-Indigenous ones, and Indigenous Peoples register higher rates for cardiovascular and respiratory diseases, infections, HIV/AIDS, malaria, cancer and malnutrition (Pan American Health Organisation, 2002; UN-DESA, 2018). The 2009 State of the World's Indigenous Peoples shows that Indigenous Peoples are more likely to experience a reduced quality of life when compared to Western standards. This is due to the high correlation between ethnicity and extreme poverty rates, the lack of access and usufruct to infrastructure and basic services and lack of targeted policies and investment (Ibidem). Indeed, life expectancy among Indigenous Peoples globally is estimated to be up to 25 years lower than non-Indigenous populations (UN-DESA, 2009).

In 2020, the legacy of extreme vulnerability resulting from exclusion and marginalisation has become evident in the impacts of climate change and natural hazards, including disease outbreak. With the COVID-19 pandemic, Indigenous Peoples' precarious livelihood and well-being have been aggravated (UN-DESA, 2020). The economic recession and the mobility restrictions worsened income stability and the already poor access to health services, water, food and sanitation systems (Ibidem). To address this urgent situation and provide accurate information on proper care, states were invited to work together with traditional healers and medicine to approach livelihood, illness and recovery in a way that respected Indigenous Peoples' culture and organisation (FAO, 2020).

Indigenous Peoples' health status cannot be separated from the devaluation and dismantling of their knowledge systems, which include medicinal practices and resource management. The deep connection Indigenous Peoples have with their environment is strictly related to their conceptualisation of health. The Western health system tends to see illness as a biological incident with poor or no relation to the social and ecological environment and as a result often promotes pharmacological solutions that seek immediate symptom relief (Meza-Calfunao et al., 2018).

Indigenous Peoples' health concept is inseparable from socio-political harmony, food systems, cosmovision and ecological well-being. Despite the wide variety in regional, country, cultural, traditional and historical contexts, (nearly all) Indigenous Peoples share a conceptualisation of health, in which health is conceptualised not as an individual factor but holistically. It is deeply connected with the land, which is not seen as private property. The health concept includes the physical and mental as well as the spiritual, social and ecological dimensions (Janska, 2008; Loncon, 2023).

In other words, the person is not separated and independent from the social and ecological environment. Rather, health equilibrium is in the interconnection and interdependence among these elements. Therefore, solutions to illness are multifaceted and expanded. They are devised to take into consideration the person's unique characteristics (from their constitution to their social environment) and to restore this balance (Janska, 2008; Meza-Calfunao et al., 2018). For example, in the Mapuche health system, discussed by Meza-Calfunao et al. (2018), the kütran (illness or spiritual imbalance, extended to family and community) is determined by an imbalance between the che (person) and the itro fill mogen (biodiversity, environment). The mapu kütran is a manifestation of illness with no apparent cause that is determined by transgressing or abusing the environment without the permission of its guardian spirit (ngen). Then, balance as a way of promoting küme mogen (good life, good living) implies that human health departs from a horizontal relationship with the natural environment, taking only what is essentially needed to maintain health and harmony (Loncon, 2023).[6] The following case study introduces some efforts towards the development of intercultural approaches to health and care.

Case Study: Intercultural Care Practices Combining Indigenous and Non-Indigenous Knowledge and Health Systems

Instead of assimilatory mechanisms, some countries are developing an intercultural approach that would combine Indigenous and non-Indigenous medical systems. As a practical example, we refer to Mignone and colleagues' work called "Best practices in intercultural health: five case studies in Latin America" (2007), where the authors compare five case studies from Chile, Colombia, Suriname, Ecuador and Guatemala. The article provides a good framework for understanding some of the benefits and difficulties of developing intercultural health care systems. One of the most interesting takeaways is that each country has developed different expressions of interculturality. Therefore, interculturality should not be reduced to one model. All of them have tried to combine the Indigenous and the Western system at all levels of organisation with the active participation of Indigenous entities. Among the most recognised opportunities are: the integration of knowledge between both types of practitioners, the increase of trust among community members towards the health care system and the increase of inclusion and active participation of Indigenous communities in decision- and policy-making.

In general terms, "the revaluing of traditional knowledge and practices and the increased sense of ownership and control over the health system appear to provide a wide range of potential benefits to indigenous communities" (Ibid.:7). Importantly, Mignone and colleagues found that barriers to access were reduced – and patients' satisfaction increased – when the intercultural health services were articulated in respect to Indigenous cosmovision and needs and when Indigenous entities were involved in their organisation. The most positive impact of these experiences was seen in increased community involvement, which in turn reflected a bettering of other health indicators such as nutritional status and employment (Ibid.:8).

Unfortunately, this aim is rarely fully achieved due to widespread Western-colonial institutionalised racism within the health care system (Ibid.:6). Furthermore, Mignone and colleagues observed varying degrees of resistance from religious sectors, especially Christianity and evangelical. In general, this poor receptivity limited the effectiveness of the services. The poor implementation and monitoring that should be guaranteed by state and other institutional actors was complicated by the lack of clear legal frameworks and regulations and by insecure funding, which subjected intercultural programs to the disposition of changing governments and economic fluctuations.

Common Violations of Indigenous Peoples' Rights

Discrimination against Indigenous Peoples is evident in the lack of recognition in constitutions or specific laws by nation-states and individuals, denying their identity, cultural heritage, protection and right to self-determination and governance of their territories. Overall, the picture that is laid in front of our eyes, one crafted also through years of fieldwork, illustrates how the colonial racism perpetuated against Indigenous Peoples underlies the most significant violations of human rights and shows all the different forms it can take. This racism, deeply entrenched in society, is perpetuated by nation-states, private corporations and individuals perpetuating white supremacism.

As mentioned before, a crucial aspect of Indigenous Peoples' rights is self-determination, encompassing land, culture and collective personhood. This right acknowledges their unique collective identity and their right to freely determine their political status and pursue economic, social and cultural development in their own ways. However, the violation of self-determination has been prevalent since colonisation, with governments and private entities often seizing Indigenous lands without their consent, leading to forced displacement and cultural erosion. Without recognition and implementation of their land rights by nation-states, Indigenous communities are vulnerable to land grabs, forced displacement and exploitation of natural resources without their consent. Indigenous communities struggle to seek redress for land disputes, environmental degradation, cultural appropriation and other injustices.

Intertwined with the violation of recognition, the denial of self-determination is manifested as political marginalisation, limiting Indigenous peoples' voice in decisions affecting them. Addressing these pervasive violations demands a steadfast commitment to recognising Indigenous People's unique cultural heritage and ensuring their active participation in decisions affecting them (Colchester, 2004; Van Cott, 2010). They are often excluded from political processes and decision-making structures, deepening their social and economic marginalisation. Additionally, Indigenous Peoples often face discrimination and marginalisation in accessing basic services such as health care, education and social welfare.

Concluding Remarks

In this chapter, we have highlighted key moments in the development of Indigenous Peoples' rights, a unique codification born out of the modern global history of European colonialism and white supremacy. The late codification of Indigenous Peoples' rights responds to Eurocentric conceptualisations of what it means to be human and live in dignity. Against the widespread human rights narrative of universalism, populations have been treated differently to privilege the energetic and economic interests of certain populations and states over others.

The erasure of historical narratives of Indigenous Peoples' Rights has contributed to a widespread ignorance that hinders the understanding of the complex and nuanced history of these communities. The consequences of such historical oversights reverberate in current societal dynamics, perpetuating systemic violence that continues to marginalise, oppress and harm Indigenous Peoples and their livelihoods. By acknowledging the injustices of the past, society can move towards tangible reparatory actions. In essence, the inclusion of Indigenous Peoples' human rights and the acknowledgment of historical injustices in educational curricula are pivotal for fostering a more just and equitable society. Only through comprehensive education and a commitment to reparative actions can we hope to break the cycle of historical mistakes and work towards building a more inclusive and respectful future for all, aligning with the principles set forth by the UN Convention.

At the international level, Global North countries (often ex-colonisers or settler colonies) benefit from the underdevelopment of Global South countries. However, in settler colonies such as the US, Australia and many Latin American countries, this disparity is also evident at the intra-national level, with dominant settler politics and culture seeking to first exterminate then assimilate Indigenous Populations out of their ancestral lands, customs and societal organisation.

The trajectory of Indigenous Peoples as subjects of rights has therefore been informed by the economic and energetic needs of coloniser countries. Until recently, Indigenous Peoples were loosely recognised, transitioning from being exterminated to being a "problem" to solve, usually through assimilation policies. The 2007 codification represents a remarkable shift: it elaborates Indigenous Peoples as a unique collective subject by drawing on the connections among well-being, knowledge systems, ecosystems and community as interdependent.

The 2007 Declaration asserts that Indigenous Peoples' rights, including their right to health, cannot be upheld without simultaneous guarantees of self-determination, collective land ownership and social policies oriented towards reducing systemic marginalisation. By recognising historical harm, the Declaration calls for strong reparative action to be executed at the state level. However, the Declaration and its call for action remain non-binding for states, which often do not implement these rights and continue to perpetuate violence originated during conquest and ongoing colonialism. Again, part of the problem is that human rights tools require states to self-regulate and to implement Indigenous rights in real life.

Questions for Discussion

■ Discuss why and how Indigenous Peoples' rights are not recognised by nation-states.
■ Discuss what is needed to reduce social marginalisation amongst Indigenous Peoples.
■ Discuss reparative measures states should implement to ensure Indigenous Peoples Rights.
■ Think about the intersectionality of the historical-ongoing colonialism and white supremacy affecting Indigenous Peoples' right in terms of recognition, culture, knowledge and cosmovision. If it applies, you can discuss the country wherein you are currently studying.
■ Discuss your perspectives on intercultural practices of (health) care.

Notes

1 It is important to note that many scholars of colonialism have highlighted how territorial names and classification are in themselves colonial operations that centre Europe (also called eurocentrism) and its political framework.
2 We refer to the extensive work of Sylvia Wynter for further discussion.
3 McHugh (2004) and Hughes (2006) discuss how some forms of recognition were developed in African territories as well, albeit with important differences.
4 Wynter (2003) elaborates how this definition of the human through a framework of rationality will shift, in the 18th and 19th centuries, into one of biological evolution and economic selection mostly through racial terms and contemporary understandings of human biological and social development, where white European countries are placed at the forefront of progress as expression of natural evolution.
5 See, for instance, the US retractions in the 19th and 20th century, discussed by Shelton, 2020.
6 Another relevant example of communal and holistic health worldview is Ubuntu, a philosophy and ethics of life, common good and health where to be and becoming human are possible only within and through the community.

References

Anaya, S. J. (2004). International human rights and indigenous peoples: The move toward the multicultural state. *Arizona Journal of International and Comparative Law, 21,* 13.

Anaya, S. J. (2009). *International human rights and indigenous peoples: 2010.* Aspen Publishing.

Asia Indigenous Peoples Pact (AIPP), & United Nations Department for Economic and Social Affairs (UN-DESA). (2015). *Situation of the right to health of indigenous peoples.* https://www.ohchr.org/Documents/Issues/IPeoples/EMRIP/Health/AIPP.pdf

Colchester, M. (2004). Conservation policy and indigenous peoples. *Environmental Science & Policy, 7*(3), 145–153.

Cox, A. (2017). *Settler colonialism.* Oxford University Press.

de Vitoria, F. (1917). *De Indis et de ivre belli relectiones.* Carnegie Institution of Washington.

Durie, M. (2004). Understanding health and illness: Research at the interface between science and indigenous knowledge. *International Journal of Epidemiology, 33*(5), 1138–1143.

EMRIP. (2019). *Indigenous peoples' rights in the context of borders, migration and displacement: Report.* https://www.ohchr.org/EN/Issues/IPeoples/EMRIP/Pages/BordersMigrationDisplacement.aspx

Errico, S. (2006). World Bank and indigenous peoples: The operational policy on indigenous peoples (OP 4.10) between indigenous peoples rights to traditional lands and to free, prior, and informed consent. *International Journal on Minority & Group Rights, 13*, 367.

FAO. (2017). *6 ways indigenous peoples are helping the world achieve #ZeroHunger*. https://www.fao.org/indigenous-peoples/news-article/en/c/1029002/

FAO. (2020). *COVID-19 and indigenous peoples*. https://www.fao.org/3/ca9106en/CA9106EN.pdf

FAO. (n.d.). *Indigenous peoples*. https://www.fao.org/indigenous-peoples/en/

Gocke, K. (2013). *Indigenous peoples in international law*. http://books.openedition.org/gup/pdf/163

Hughes, L. (2006). *Moving the Maasai: A colonial misadventure*. Palgrave Macmillan.

IACHR. (2000). *The human rights situation of the indigenous people in the Americas. Chapter 1: Historical background of the rights of indigenous people under the Inter-American System.* (OAS Doc. OEA/Ser.L/V/II.108, Doc. 62). https://cidh.oas.org/Indigenas/chap.1.htm

IACHR. (2017). *Towards effective integral protection policies for human rights defenders*. http://www.oas.org/en/iachr/reports/pdfs/Defensores-eng-2017.pdf

ILO. (2003). *Indigenous and tribal peoples convention, 1989* (No. 169). ILO.

Inter-American Development Bank. (1997). *Annual report 1997*. Inter-American Development Bank. www.iadb.org

IWGIA. (2019). *International year of indigenous languages*. www.iwgia.org/en/news/3302-year-of-indigenous-languages.html

Janska, E. (2008). Health knowledge, traditional. In W. Kirch (Ed.), *Encyclopedia of public health*. Springer.

Jones, P. (2016, Summer). Group rights. In E. N. Zalta (Ed.), *The Stanford encyclopedia of philosophy*. https://plato.stanford.edu/archives/sum2016/entries/rights-group/

Loncon, E. (2023). *Az Mapu: Aportes de la filosofía Mapuche para el cuidado del lof y la madre tierra*. Ariel (Ed).

MacKay, F. (2005). The draft World Bank operational policy 4.10 on indigenous peoples: Progress or more of the same. *Arizona Journal of International and Comparative Law, 22*, 65.

Malezer, L. (2005). Permanent forum on indigenous issues: "Welcome to the family of the UN". In *International law and indigenous peoples* (pp. 67–86). Brill Nijhoff.

McHugh, P. G. (2004). *Aboriginal societies and the common law: A history of sovereignty, status, and self-determination*. Oxford University Press.

Meza-Calfunao, E., Díaz-Fuentes, R., & Alarcón-Muñoz, A. M. (2018). ¿Qué es küme mogen mapuche? Concepto e implicancias en salud pública y comunitaria. *Salud pública de México, 60*, 380–381.

Mignone, J., Bartlett, J., O'Neil, J., & Orchard, T. (2007). Best practices in intercultural health: Five case studies in Latin America. *Journal of Ethnobiology and Ethnomedicine, 3*(1), 1–11.

Ohenjo, N., Willis, R., Jackson, D., Nettleton, C., Good, K., & Mugarura, B. (2006). Indigenous health in Africa. *Lancet, 367*(10).

Pan American Health Organisation. (2002). *Health in the Americas*. www.paho.org

Quijano, A. (2000). Coloniality of power and Eurocentrism in Latin America. *International Sociology, 15*(2), 215–232.

Ring, I., & Brown, N. (2003). The health status of indigenous peoples and others. *BMJ, 327*(7412), 404–405.

Rivera-Cusicanqui, S. (2010). *Ch'ixinakax utxiwa: una reflexión sobre prácticas y discursos descolonizadores*. Tinta Limón (Ed).

Rodney, W. (2018). *How Europe underdeveloped Africa*. Verso Books.

Samson, C. (2020). *The colonialism of human rights: Ongoing hypocrisies of western liberalism*. John Wiley & Sons.

Shelton, D. (2020). The rights of indigenous peoples: Everything old is new again. In A. von Arnauld, K. von der Decken, & M. Susi (Eds.), *The Cambridge handbook of new human rights: Recognition, novelty, rhetoric* (pp. 217–232). Cambridge University Press.

Singel, W. T. (2008). New directions for international law and indigenous peoples. *Idaho Law Review*, 45, 509.

Swepston, L. (2015). The foundations of modern international law on indigenous and tribal peoples: The preparatory documents of the indigenous and tribal peoples convention, and its development through supervision. Vol. 1: Basic policy and land rights. In *The foundations of modern international law on indigenous and tribal peoples*. Brill Nijhoff.

UN. (2006). *The Millenium development goals and indigenous peoples*. un.org/esa/socdev/unpfii/documents/5session_factsheet2.pdf

UN. (2007). *United Nations declaration on the rights of indigenous peoples*. https://www.un.org/development/desa/indigenouspeoples/wpcontent/uploads/sites/19/2018/11/UNDRIP_E_web.pdf

UN DESA. (2009). *State of the world's indigenous peoples*. https://www.un.org/esa/socdev/unpfii/documents/SOWIP/en/SOWIP_web.pdf

UN DESA. (2012). *United Nations declaration on the rights of indigenous peoples*. https://www.un.org/development/desa/indigenouspeoples/declaration-on-the-rights-of-indigenouspeoples.html

UN DESA. (2018). *State of the world's indigenous peoples*. https://www.un.org/development/desa/indigenouspeoples/wp-content/uploads/sites/19/2018/03/TheState-of-The-Worlds-Indigenous-Peoples-WEB.pdf

UN DESA. (2020). *Indigenous peoples and the COVID-19 pandemic: Considerations*. https://www.un.org/development/desa/indigenouspeoples/wp-content/uploads/sites/19/2020/04/COVID19_IP_considerations.pdf

Van Cott, D. L. (2010). Indigenous peoples' politics in Latin America. *Annual Review of Political Science*, 13, 385–405.

Veracini, L. (2010). *Settler colonialism*. Palgrave Macmillan.

Veracini, L. (2013). "Settler colonialism": Career of a concept. *The Journal of Imperial and Commonwealth History*, 41(2), 313–333.

World Bank Organization. (2020). *Indigenous peoples*. https://www.worldbank.org/en/topic/indigenouspeoples

World Health Organization. (2007). *The health of indigenous peoples – fact sheet*. https://www.who.int/gender-equity-rights/knowledge/factsheet-indigenous-healthn-nov2007-eng.pdf

Wynter, S. (2003). Unsettling the coloniality of being/power/truth/freedom: Towards the human, after man, its overrepresentation – an argument. *CR: The New Centennial Review*, 3(3), 257–337.

Future Challenges in Global Health and Human Rights

In this third part, we focus on developments that will pose serious challenges to the delivery of health care and to the management of health care systems. This is obviously a very tall order as the common future of humanity is challenged by multiple worrisome trends. Among them are growing economic disparities and social exclusivism, non-democratic movements and shrinking spaces for cultural innovation. Gostin and Meier (2020) also highlight challenges arising from international trade and radical right-wing populism.

Climate change – or, more positively framed, "planetary health" – is another contemporary issue in health and human rights which poses significant challenges to the future of health, food security and human rights. Clearly, human and planetary health are intertwined; humans need breathable air, drinkable water and edible food. But, additionally, climate change may result in death and illness due to the growing frequency of extreme weather events, such as heatwaves, storms and floods. It can also disrupt food systems, increase the prevalence of zoonotic diseases and spread food-, water- and vector-borne diseases, while these events may contributing to mental health distress. These linkages are acknowledged by the global community. In July 2022, the UN General Assembly recognised the "right to a clean, healthy and sustainable environment as a human right" (Resolution A/76/L.75).

The future of food security – the right to food – is also a crosscutting contemporary and future challenge that affects the right to health directly and indirectly. In 2022, over 900 million people were food insecure; there were 2.5 billion adults who were overweight, including 890 million who were living with obesity, while 390 million adults were underweight. Additionally, on a global scale, it was estimated that 149 million children under the age of 5 were stunted (too short for their age), 45 million were wasted (too thin for their height) and 37 million were either overweight or living with obesity. Today, half of all childhood deaths are related to malnutrition. These figures are likely to become worse as food prices keep on rising, climate change severely affects agriculture and the sector itself needs change as the global agrifood system contributes

DOI: 10.4324/9781003408765-14

almost one-third of all greenhouse gas emissions worldwide. The right to health will be increasingly challenged as nutrition-related illness will demand more resources from already stretched health systems. In particular, in low- and middle-income countries many health systems have only recently adapted to the challenges of the increasing rise of Non-Communicable Diseases (NCDs). NCDs, such as diabetes, cancer and cardio-vascular diseases, require a different approach than dealing with more acute illness. For example, it requires continuity of care – including continuous access to diagnostics and medicine – at multiple levels of the health system from specialised inpatient care to the management of self-care in household settings.

In 2024 the International Rescue Committee stated that a great and dangerous challenge to the right to health is posed by the world's humanitarian crises. These include armed conflicts and the worldwide forced displacements (by the end of 2023, more than 114 million people) as a result of persecution, conflict, violence or human rights violations. These displacements include (35.3 million) refugees, (62.5 million) internally displaced people, (5.4 million) asylum seekers and (5.2 million) people in need of international protection. In 2024, the International Rescue Committee listed 20 countries in which people were at great risk of a crisis of spreading diseases; shortages of medical supplies and nutritional aid; insufficient access to medical services, clean water and sanitation and the permanent threat of murder, torture and rape.

Among all these challenges and risks we have chosen to focus on the themes of global infectious diseases and advances in medical technology. These themes encapsulate immediate threats and long-term opportunities in global health and human rights, which can be transformative for the future of human rights-based health care, making them pivotal areas for discussion. The conclusion of Part III, as the final chapter of the book, introduces a guide designed to help students critically think about and plan for the future of human rights-based health care. This guide aims to support future practitioners to navigate and address the evolving landscape of global health and human rights challenges.

References

Bostrom, N., & Cirković, M. M. (2008). *Global catastrophic risks*. Oxford University Press. Future Healthcare Journal (open access). Editor in chief, Andrew Duncombe, University Hospital Southampton NHS Foundation Trust, Southampton, United Kingdom.

Gostin, L. O., & Meier, B. M. (2020). *Foundations of global health & human rights*. Oxford University Press, Section Four New Challenges.

Public Health Emergencies, Pandemics and Human Rights

Dirk R. Essink

Introduction

Can we rob individuals of their rights just because they are sick? Or when we suspect them to be sick? Or when we suspect their day-to-day behaviour may increase disease transmission? How can we make decisions with increasing uncertainty? Are warlike rhetorics that are often used to address infectious diseases, like in "the fight against COVID", not contradicting the very nature of human rights? In this chapter we discuss these fundamental questions in the context of public health emergencies of international concern (PHEIC). Whilst most chapters of this book take the right to health of the individual as a starting point, this chapter considers the right to health (and security) of the public. For instance, we consider to what extent – if at all – the rights of an individual can be compromised to improve or protect public health. This is a true dilemma concretely highlighted by the recent COVID-19 outbreak.

For centuries, governments have implemented policies to curb the spread of infectious diseases and to reduce related infections, illness and death. However, these measures have often infringed on the rights of individuals. For example, isolation of infected individuals, quarantining those suspected of infection, prohibiting public/social gatherings and restricting visitors to private homes are at odds with people's right to freedom in public and private spheres and their right to mobility. Other possible measures, such as mandatory testing and mandatory vaccination, may challenge individual bodily integrity and autonomy. These interventions are subject to scrutiny, especially when one considers the difficulties in attributing fault to individuals for becoming infected. This raises critical questions: how dangerous must an infection be to justify imposing such measures? And what criteria should guide decisions on the implementation of interventions? These issues will be explored in this chapter.

DOI: 10.4324/9781003408765-15

Learning Objectives

After studying this chapter you will be able to:

- Understand the International Health Regulations
- Understand the principles of limitation and derogation in relation to the International Health Regulations and infectious diseases outbreaks
- Identify common human rights infringements during infectious disease outbreaks
- Discuss human rights during the COVID-19 pandemic.

The Legal Framework: The International Health Regulations

In 2007, Margaret Chan as Director General of the WHO stated that, within contemporary global society, characterised by high mobility, economic interdependence and environmental degradation, infectious diseases represent one of the most serious health dangers to humanity (Heymann et al., 2007). Infectious agents spread fast and may affect many individuals directly and indirectly. The consequences can be devastating. This is not and has never been a hypothetical threat. We have experienced the consequences of COVID-19, just as societies before us have experienced the bubonic plague, the "Spanish Flu", SARS and many others.

The International Covenant on Economic, Social and Cultural Rights already emphasised that epidemic prevention and response is at the core of Article 12 on the right to health. In 1969 the UN World Health Assembly first adopted the International Health Regulations (IHR). The IHR are a legally binding instrument of international law and should be understood in conjunction with the ICESCR. The principle aim of this instrument is "to prevent, protect against, control, and provide a public health response to the international spread of disease in ways that are commensurate with and restricted to public health risks and that avoid unnecessary interference with international traffic and trade". After the lessons learned from the SARS outbreak, the IHR were revised and reconfirmed in 2007 (WHO, 2008).

In addition to retaining its focus on vectors, diseases and sanitary measures for ships, aircraft, ports and airports, the IHR 2005 introduces several new elements, including: i) a scope not limited to any specific disease or manner of transmission but covering "illness or medical condition, irrespective of origin or source, that presents or could present significant harm to humans"; ii) state party obligations to develop certain minimum core public health capacities; iii) obligations on States Parties to notify the WHO of events that may constitute a public health emergency of international concern according to defined criteria; iv) provisions authorising the WHO to take into consideration unofficial reports of public health events and to obtain verification from States Parties concerning such events; v) procedures for the determination by the director general of a "public health emergency of international concern" and issuance of corresponding temporary recommendations, after taking into account the views of an Emergency Committee; (vi) protection of the human rights of persons and travellers; and (vii) the establishment of National IHR Focal Points and WHO IHR Contact Points for urgent communications between States Parties and the WHO (WHO, 2008).

In total, 196 countries have adopted the IHR, recognising that certain public health incidents need to be designated as a Public Health Emergency of International Concern (PHEIC). Countries thereby commit themselves to monitoring and surveillance and taking appropriate action. If two of the following four questions are confirmed, then a potential PHEIC exists and the WHO should be notified:

- Is the public health impact of the event serious?
- Is the event unusual or unexpected?
- Is there a significant risk of international spread?
- Is there a significant risk for international travel or trade restrictions?

Since the adoption of the IHR 2005, the WHO has declared a PHEIC on seven different occasions (see Textbox 11.1). However, recent studies have identified that there is lack of consistency in the application of criteria to determine a PHEIC as defined by the IHR (Mullen et al., 2020).

Textbox 11.1
PHEIC Since the Adoption of the IHR (2005)

- 2009–2010 H1N1 (or swine flu) pandemic
- The 2013–2016 outbreak of Ebola in Western Africa
- The 2015–2016 Zika virus epidemic
- The 2018–2020 Kivu Ebola epidemic
- The 2020–2023 declaration for the COVID-19 pandemic
- The 2022–2023 mpox outbreak
- The 2014-ongoing polio outbreak/eradication

Additionally, severe acute respiratory syndrome (SARS), smallpox, wild type poliomyelitis and new subtypes of human influenza are considered PHEIC per default.

Although the IHR are internationally accepted and the director general of the WHO can declare a PHEIC, sovereign states are accountable and responsible for their implementation. As such, countries have adopted national laws derived from the IHR within their respective legal frameworks. The IHR – and their national derivatives – form a legally binding instrument that enables sovereign states to take actions that may compromise the rights of individuals to protect the health of the public and the functioning of the states in public health emergencies. Concurrently, the IHR also mandates states to be prepared. For example, in Article 18 of the IHR, "Recommendations with respect to persons, baggage, cargo, containers, conveyances, goods and postal parcels", it is stated amongst other points (see Textbox 11.1) that quarantine and isolation may be imposed on individuals, and medical screening may be applied. However, such stringent measures can only be implemented when a country is confronted with a public health emergency. The IHR also provides a decision tool to identify when an event can be considered as such. A closer examination of this tool makes apparent that such events are likely to be rare. The IHR also state that countries need to be prepared, referring to the need to build capacity for the implementation of the IHR. This includes – but is not limited to – surveillance systems and ensuring capacity for implementation of measures.

Furthermore – and arguably most important for this chapter – the IHR explicitly states that measures should always respect the human rights of individuals and be compatible with the international human rights standards. This is articulated in the foreword, as well as in Articles 3 and 32. Article 3 states, "the implementation of these Regulations shall be with full respect for the dignity, human rights and fundamental freedoms of persons". Article 32 specifically addresses the rights of travellers, stating "In implementing health measures under these Regulations, States Parties shall treat travellers with respect for their dignity, human rights and fundamental freedoms and minimise any discomfort or distress associated with such measures". However, few rigorous evaluations of human rights violations have been conducted during or following the following PHEIC (Bennett & Carney, 2017). It is evident that human rights violations have occurred during such emergencies. For example, during the recent COVID-19 pandemic, the Human Rights Measurement Initiative clearly stated that "2020 was not a good year for civil and political rights and for social and economic rights". For example, violations included restrictions on freedom of assembly and demonstration and on the right to work, and in most countries migrants and marginalised groups were the ones disproportionately impacted. Determining violations of the right to health during PHEICs (Textbox 11.1) is more complex, as these emergencies are primarily declared to safeguard public health. Nevertheless, such measures often come at a cost; for example, access to general health and preventive services was significantly hindered during the Ebola outbreaks in West Africa and the Congo. Later in this chapter we will look at this more specifically using the case of the COVID-19 outbreak.

A closer examination of national applications of the IHR shows different approaches in relation to human rights. In China, the Law on the Prevention and Control of Infectious Diseases (2013) provides the legal framework for managing infectious diseases, including measures for surveillance, prevention, control and response to outbreaks. Notably, measures that may be enforced on patients include isolation, quarantine and treatment, whereas in the Dutch Public Health Act we can observe that on the one hand public health emergencies allow for infringement of certain individual rights, but at the same time the individual is safeguarded as severe measurements may only be applied in rare cases (van Vliet, 2009). For example, in the Netherlands, home isolation and medical examination may only be forced upon people when there is a (suspected) case of Group A notifiable diseases, and treatment can never be enforced. Furthermore, judicial review has to take place within days to justify any measures imposed on the individual(s). Ultimately, local or national authorities are responsible for implementing measures against infectious disease outbreaks. However, the public health acts do stipulate the establishment of specified expert teams to advise decisions makers.

Besides the IHR and national derivatives, governments have additional laws that can be used to implement and enforce measures that limit the protection of rights of individuals, most notably laws that allow for declaring a situation a national emergency. For example, in Spain and the US, COVID-19 was declared an emergency situation. Furthermore, governments may formulate laws that are specifically addressing an outbreak. For example, China formulated its "zero-COVID" policy at the start of the outbreak, and the Netherlands adopted the "Corona law" on 27 October 2020.

Thus, by international and national law, the right to freedom and integrity of the body of individuals may be rendered inferior to the right to security of the population.

Bear in mind that these individuals at this point have not clearly done something wrong prior to the limiting of these individual rights. They may just happen to be sick, or they may be suspected of being sick.

Amendments to the IHR 2024 and Pandemic Agreement

In response to the COVD-19 pandemic, WHO working groups have concurrently been developing amendments to the IHR and a Pandemic Agreement. Both instruments aim to enhance global capacity and coordination in addressing health emergencies, such as outbreaks and pandemics. However, the Pandemic Agreement has a narrower scope and is regarded as a "Treaty" and thus carries more binding obligations for states. On 28 May 2024, the World Health Assembly agreed upon amendments to the IHR. Negotiations on a Pandemic Agreement were extended by up to one year.

The amendments to the IHR provide a definition for "pandemic" and introduce an additional classification of "pandemic emergency" as a specific type PHEIC that can be declared by the director general of the WHO. It enables the director general to issue an "early action alert", which offers information and non-binding advice to member states about a health event that does not yet meet the criteria for a PHEIC. Additionally, the amendments highlight the importance of solidarity and equity in accessing medical products and financing by establishing a Coordinating Financial Mechanism. This mechanism aims to assist countries in securing the necessary funding to meet their needs and priorities in pandemic prevention, preparedness and response. The amendments also aim to enhance compliance and implementation by requiring Member States to establish a "National IHR Authority" responsible for coordinating the implementation of IHR requirements within the country, in addition to the already established National Focal Point. Additionally, provisions are made to create an "Implementation and Compliance Committee" to facilitate and oversee the implementation of – and promote compliance with – the IHR.

While the amendments address vaccine inequalities and emphasise solidarity between countries, they do not explicitly promote human rights. On the contrary, executive power to promote public health may be expanded by the amendments to the IHR and potential Pandemic Agreements, which could, in turn, compromise human rights. For example, both the IHR and the Pandemic Agreement aim to enhance the WHO's emergency and bio-surveillance powers, strengthen countries' capacities for disease surveillance and notifications and facilitate access to emergency medical technology. Although these measures can promote public health security, they might also breach confidentiality, reduce the safety of medical products and enforce measures that unjustly compromise individual rights.

Limitations and Derogations

As stated previously, the IHR explicitly state that there are situations in which the rights of persons may be affected (Murphy, 2013). Therefore, in such instances, human rights considerations should be incorporated into the decision-making process. This implies that it should be compatible with the human rights standards; the moral code of our international community. Zidar (2015) portrays how two different approaches may be taken to justify any incursions in human rights: the "limitations" and the "derogations" models. As its name suggests, the limitation model limits the protection of human rights. The derogations model temporarily suspends the rights, except for core rights that may never be reduced or detracted from. With regard to limitations, the UDHR included that limitations "are determined by law solely for the purpose of securing due recognition and respect for the rights and freedoms of others and of meeting the just requirements of morality, public order and the general welfare in a democratic society". The Siracusa Principles on the Limitation and Derogation of Provisions in the ICCPR of 1984 explicitly stated that public health threats may form a legitimate reason for states to limit the protection of human rights. Any limitations should prevent disease or provide care for the sick and should take into account proportionality. In the Siracusa Principles paragraph 10, it is further stated that any limitation must further comply with the following criteria: i) it must be based on one of the grounds justifying limitations (that is, public health); ii) it must respond to a pressing public or social need; iii) it must pursue a legitimate aim and iv) it must be proportionate to that aim (UN, 1984; Upshur, 2002).

The derogations model is far less balanced than the limitations model. In essence, it enables states to detract from the protection of human rights on the basis of an emergency. The Siracusa Principles state that a threat to the life of the nation must be a situation of exceptional and actual or imminent danger that: i) affects the whole of the population and the whole or part of the territory of the state and ii) threatens the physical integrity of the population, the political independence or the territorial integrity of the state or the existence or basic functioning of institutions indispensable for the protection of rights. However, there are a limited number of human rights provisions from which no derogation is possible – not even in a state of national emergency. These are mentioned in Article 4 of the ICCPR. No derogation is permitted from Articles 6, 7, 8 (paragraphs I and 2), 11, 15, 16 and 18, not even in times of a public emergency which threatens the existence of the nation. They include the inherent right to life, the right not to be subjected to torture or to cruel, inhuman or degrading treatment or punishment and the right to freedom of thought, conscience and religion.

But when and how do we define something as an emergency? The IHR outline a process for declaring emergencies that includes specific criteria for notifiable diseases, while also allowing sufficient flexibility to address unusual and unforeseen events. Simultaneously, the Siracusa Principles offer additional points on identifying emergencies and implementing appropriate measures: i) no limitation on a right recognised by the ICCPR shall be discriminatory; ii) any limitations must respond to a pressing public or social need, pursue a legitimate aim and be proportional to that aim; iii) states should use no more restrictive means than are required for the achievement of the purpose of the limitation; iv) the burden of justifying a limitation upon a right guaranteed under the ICCPR lies with the state; and v) every limitation imposed shall be subject to the possibility of challenge to and remedy against its abusive application.

Human Rights in a Pandemic, PHEIC: Common Violations and Controversies

The complexities become more profound when we zoom in on some of the difficult choices to make. During a pandemic, the right to privacy, liberty and the freedom of individuals are at stake. But inaction may also compromise the life and livelihoods of the public. This is the clearest controversy and any decision should be made with proportionality in mind. For example, the right to privacy – encompassing identity, integrity, intimacy, autonomy, communication and sexuality – is at odds with many measures that are part of the IHR Article 18 (see Textbox 11.2). Some are more directly linked to privacy, such as: the review of the travel history, the review of proof of medical examination, laboratory analysis and the tracing of contacts. Others more severely affect the integrity and autonomy of individuals, the requirement to undergo medical examination – which may include physical examination – and the requirement of vaccination or other prophylaxis.

Textbox 11.2
Extract of Part One of Article 18 of the IHR

Recommendations issued by the WHO to States Parties with respect to persons may include the following advice:

- No specific health measures are advised
- Review travel history in affected areas
- Review proof of medical examination and any laboratory analysis
- Require medical examinations
- Review proof of vaccination or other prophylaxis
- Require vaccination or other prophylaxis
- Place suspect persons under public health observation
- Implement quarantine or other health measures for suspect persons
- Implement isolation and treatment where necessary of affected persons
- Implement tracing of contacts of suspect or affected persons
- Refuse entry of suspect and affected persons
- Refuse entry of unaffected persons to affected areas and implement exit screening and/ or restrictions on persons from affected areas.

The right to liberty is profoundly affected by the placement of suspect persons under public health observation, the imposition of a quarantine or other similar health measures for suspect persons and the submission of affected persons to isolation and treatment where necessary. Furthermore, Article 18 of the IHR severely affects the freedom of movement. For example, states may refuse entry of suspected and affected persons, refuse entry of unaffected persons to affected areas and implement exit screening and/ or restrictions on persons from affected areas. The IHR further stipulate that, on a routine basis, states may require individuals entering the country to be vaccinated. On a more abstract level, the ICESR and the IHR stipulate that governments should be prepared to address epidemics. The lack of preparedness can be considered a human rights violation on its own account.

Furthermore, epidemics affect groups disproportionally, and most responses are not tailored to vulnerable groups, leading to (persisting) inequalities. For example, Stemple and colleagues (2016), show how gender norms – not biology – lead to women being more affected by HIV/AIDS and Ebola and how responses to epidemics may increase risk of gender based violence. Davies and Bennett (2016) show that responses to Zika and Ebola ignored that prevailing gender norms (e.g., wrongly assuming women could take autonomous actions) further compounded inequalities between men and women.

Also, ethnic minorities, drug users and the LGBTQI+ communities are often more affected by outbreaks and/or the related responses.

Adding another layer of complexity, we need to assess potential benefits and harms of limiting individual rights. First of all, the assumed benefits are often described in infections adverted, reduced morbidity and reduced mortality. Benefits are generally also enlarged to economic gains, such as the costs for treatment and the loss of productivity of those affected. However, when measures are applied on a large scale, as was the case with the COVID-19 pandemic, the harms of these actions are also felt at the population level. For example, extensive quarantine measures negatively impacted the mental health of those in quarantine and significantly affected state economies, resulting in high unemployment. Other relevant question concern who is affected by the outbreak and who can make the decisions.

Decision-making When Faced with Uncertainty

The acute nature of PHEIC, the lack of evidence on effectiveness of interventions and the aforementioned trade-offs between actions to curb pandemics – the right to security of the many – and human rights of individuals demonstrate the complexity of decision-making during PHEIC. Pandemics – like many other social issues – are non-linear phenomena, where even a minor disruption within a system can lead to exponential, disproportionate reactions. In other words, both the outbreak and how we deal with it are the outcome of a complex adaptive system (CAS), the combination of many heterogeneous, interacting and adaptive agents (Angeli & Montefusco, 2020). These aspects characterise both disease spread and containment policies, resulting in unpredictable outcomes, highly dependent on context and behaviours, governing organisations and individuals (e.g., Greenhalgh, 2020; Angeli & Montefusco, 2020). Understanding how agents influence each other becomes quintessential. On a global scale, the past Covid outbreak echoed the diverse and unpredictable responses. For example, compliance of human beings in relation to measures differed across and within countries, emphasising that the human species is largely guided by cultural and social cues. To illustrate, COVID-19 vaccination acceptance was as low as 35% in Syria, compared to almost 90% in Brazil. Also, severity of lockdown policies and compliance varied across countries and is likely determined by cultural factors.

In particular, during outbreaks, the lack of evidence and consensus on the interpretation of this evidence further contributes to decision-makers' "bounded rationality" (Christensen & Mortensen, 2024). For example, critical evidence on viral transmission and disease progression is often missing at the start of an outbreak, and new mutations and changing behaviours of actors create gaps in our understanding, in particular because we as human beings are inherently social and culturally bound creatures, constrained in the ability to rationally process information about the world. With such uncertainty, decisions often focus on minimising worst outcomes. Regardless, policymakers, stakeholders and the public assign different values to potential benefits and harms of (non)interventions. Generally, they value benefits such as infections averted or reduced morbidity and mortality (e.g., Chorus, 2020). However, saving lives in the short term might sacrifice lives, social order, education and well-being in the longer term, considering the risks of economic recession and mental health consequences of prolonged lockdown and social distancing. Parameters for decision-making are ambiguous and constantly shifting, making the decision-making process inaccurate and short-sighted. This is further aggravated as decision-makers make decisions on such emergencies within the public health frame, basing their advice on insights from the (bio)medical and epidemiological experts, often excluding experts in the fields such as behavioural sciences, economics or human rights. Most PHEIC can clearly be characterised as a "wicked problem" or "unstructured problem" (Hisschemöller & Hoppe, 1995; Rittel & Webber, 1973). In dealing with such problems, a deliberative and inclusive process of learning is suggested (ibid).

So, during PHEIC/outbreaks, bounded in rationality and by time, decision-makers should be aware that policy measures thus only provide contextual solutions, applicable only within a specific timeframe. New data or unforeseen consequences may challenge assumptions, rendering previous decisions invalid. Also, decision-makers need to recognise non-linear processes and non-measurable system states, preparing for the potential of unpredictable and disproportionate outcomes resulting from their actions (Angeli & Montefusco, 2020). Human rights violations are among the most important of such outcomes. Decisions makers should therefore organise a platform with a range of stakeholders from science and society that enables rapid-cycle evaluations and (in) action inclusive of new (scientific) information. These stakeholders should include but not be limited to (public) health specialists. Additionally, in "regular" times pandemic preparedness plans should be made and practised – inclusive of rigorous human rights monitoring.

COVID-19 and Human Rights

In a brief time period, there has been a ravaging spread of the novel coronavirus disease (COVID-19) all over the world. In its spread, COVID-19 did not discriminate among nations, race/ethnicity or socioeconomic status. Its impact, however, was distributed unequally; the financially secure had, for instance, better means to protect themselves than the poor did (Ahmed et al., 2020; Smith & Judd, 2020; The Lancet Global Health, 2020; Wenham et al., 2020). There was a global focus on "flattening the curve" to reduce the surge and spread of COVID-19 cases through containment strategies that were predominantly based on border closures, lockdowns and physical distancing measures. In a short time period, epidemiological evidence for the effectiveness of such measures as a containment strategy was collected. This evidence made policy-makers and governments focus almost exclusively on preventing the immediate fatalities and effects of COVID-19. Yet, measures focusing on reducing the spread of COVID-19 alone did not capture or prevent the full societal impact of the pandemic (Landry et al., 2020). They left out the equally real but indirect effects of malnutrition, extreme poverty and lack of access to health care services for other conditions, which lockdowns or curfews aggravated (Hankivsky & Kapilashrami, 2020; Wingfield et al., 2020). This raises the question of whether the central narrative of our response to future pandemics should emphasise vigilance and solidarity in the face of a crisis or whether it should focus on the failure of many states to uphold their human rights obligations.

At the time of writing (November 2023), the WHO COVID-19 dashboard reports that worldwide there have been close to 800 million confirmed cases of COVID-19 and almost 7 million reported COVID-19 deaths, with around 13.5 billion administered vaccines. In reality, these figures were much higher. The economic and social impact of (the measures against) COVID-19 is also severe. For example, global GDP dropped 3.4% in the first 3 months of 2020 (OECD, 2020); an estimated 400 million jobs were lost between April and June 2020 (McKeever, 2020), and income of workers fell by 10% in the first 9 months of 2020. Furthermore, lockdown policies were affecting the social life and mental health of people all across the globe.

The COVID-19 pandemic is a textbook example of the conflict between individual rights and public security. Failing to act would have compromised both public health and safety. At the same time, the measures implemented to contain the virus had profound implications for the enjoyment of all human rights across populations, regardless of individual risk levels. This chapter will further explore the human rights and ethical dilemmas that emerged from the interventions enacted.

The COVID pandemic showed that the selection, allocation and impact of interventions are highly contextual; culture matters. In a global analysis by Gelfand and colleagues in the *Lancet* (2021), it was estimated that countries with high levels of cultural "looseness" (e.g., Argentina, the Netherlands, Brazil) had almost five times higher mortality rates than countries with high levels of cultural "tightness" (e.g., Vietnam, Indonesia, Saudi Arabia). This suggests that tight social norms can play a protective role during public health crises. Other studies showed that countries that exhibit collectivist cultures had lower COVID morbidity and mortality (e.g., Rajkumar, 2023; Song & Choi, 2023). For example, Song and Choi (2023) attributed the significantly higher mortality rate in the US compared to South Korea to cultural differences. They argue that public compliance with COVID measures was notably higher in South Korea, driven by a cultural emphasis on communal benefits. In contrast, the more individualistic culture in the US led to greater resistance to government policies that restricted individual freedoms.

It is argued that if a lockdown, which limits the freedom of movement, can be compatible with human rights, then compulsory vaccination might also be justified on similar grounds. However, under current laws, compulsory vaccination is generally prohibited and is considered assault if administered without consent. In the ICCPR it is stated that certain rights cannot be derogated from, including the right to be free from inhuman or degrading treatment. Mandatory vaccination conflicts with individual autonomy and bodily integrity. Compulsory interference with a person's bodily integrity is not something that a democratic society will tolerate without detailed regulations and specialist tribunals in place. A lack of mental capacity coupled with the risk to health of the individual and to the public is the only justification we have for such a draconian measure. The more pressing discussion will be regarding vaccine distribution: "who gets the vaccine (first)?" Should priority be given to groups at risk for severe disease progression or those critical in the transmission chain? Another crucial question is: "to what extent do we limit the freedoms of those who remain unvaccinated?" For instance, should unvaccinated health care workers be allowed to work with the elderly, or should unvaccinated individuals be permitted to attend large events like music concerts? The actual human rights discussion might revolve around these issues, requiring a cautious yet pragmatic approach. We must be cautious to avoid coercing people into vaccination just to participate in society, thereby preventing unnecessary discrimination. At the same time, a pragmatic approach is necessary because vaccine availability can be limited, and it is unrealistic to vaccinate everyone immediately. Balancing these concerns is essential to uphold human rights while effectively managing public health.

Much of the discourse emphasises the right to security, the right to life of the public and the rights of the individual as laid down in the ICCPR. These have been described earlier in a more abstract manner – and were already foreseen in the IHR and Siracusa Principles – such as the deprivation of freedom, privacy and liberty. Also, it has been clearly pointed out that COVID-19 policies have been used against political dissidents – governments that recently violated citizens' human rights were about 10–15% more likely to enact lockdown and curfew policies. By no means should these be trivialised; these are arguably the most significant human rights violations. However, this section highlights some of the more health-related and less well-described human rights controversies that have emerged during the pandemic that are more related to the ICESCR. For example, Article 11 of this Covenant stipulates that everybody is entitled to an adequate standard of living, explicitly mentioning food security. Furthermore, Article 12 emphasises the right to the enjoyment of the highest attainable standard of physical and mental health, which includes prevention in times of epidemics. Article 13 addresses the right to education, whilst Article 14 stipulates the right to take part in cultural activities. All of these will be discussed in more detail later. Note that this section provides examples from different parts of the world and by no means states that all violations were similar within and across countries. As indicated before, context matters in the implementation of interventions.

In relation to poverty and inequality: the Covid pandemic affected societal groups unequally. For example, in the US, Native American, Black and Latinx people had two times as high death rates from COVID-19 compared to White Americans (CDC, 2022). In 2021, the UK government announced that age-adjusted mortality rates for Pakistani and Bangladeshi British people were three to four times that of White British people. In Brazil, during the first wave, prevalence was four times higher for Indigenous populations than White Brazilian people (Gostin et al., 2023). COVID-19 was almost twice as deadly in lower-income countries (Levin et al., 2022). A study conducted in Mexico showed that the lowest income groups had a five times higher mortality rate (adjusted for co-morbidities) than the highest income group (Arceo-Gomez et al., 2022).

These inequalities can partly be explained by the containment policies that affect people in poverty disproportionately. In the case of COVID-19 lockdown policies, the poor were barred from their right to secure their livelihoods and nutrition as policies prevented people from going to work. The poor often rely on daily wage labour and lack savings to compensate. Also, they often live in densely populated areas, which may increase risk of infection in case of lockdowns – and lockdowns in such settings can easily result in the experience of humiliation. Vulnerable populations, such as migrants, people in poverty and informal workers, are even more at risk (Vieira et al., 2020). They face a higher risk for contracting and poor treatment of the disease due to overcrowding, poor nutrition, poverty and lack of access to health services. Vulnerable populations benefit less from (social) safety measures and are likely to be extraordinarily harmed by containment measures such as lockdowns (Mander, 2020). Even in countries like the Netherlands, the lockdown policies affected the poor disproportionately (Yerkes et al., 2020).

The UN interagency task force on financing for development 2022 argued that COVID-19 has pushed at least an additional 80 million people into extreme poverty. This is the first increase in global poverty since 1997, wiping out all progress made since. Particularly in LMICs, where health systems and socioeconomic conditions are commonly less resilient, pandemics exacerbate existing social and health inequities (Vieira et al., 2020; Oshitani et al., 2008). The consequences of COVID-19 are not well known yet, but the uneven distribution of effects of previous pandemics on different populations are well known (Barro et al., 2020; Phua, 2015). COVID-19 appears to be yet another disease that is a symptom of poverty.

In relation to food security: restrictions on trade and lockdown policies affected people's most basic need: food. The COVID-19 crisis aggravated the ongoing food and nutrition security crisis, contributing to the World Food Program's recognition as a Nobel Prize laureate in 2020. In April 2020, the World Food Program warned that an additional 130 million people could face acute food insecurity by the end of 2020, on top of the 135 million people who were already acutely food insecure before the crisis, due to income and remittance losses (Anthem, 2020). Six months later, the evidence on food insecurity was piling up.

In relation to education: the right to education was hampered by the suspension of in-class education in many of the COVID-19 affected countries. Almost all governments around the world temporarily closed primary, secondary and tertiary educational institutions in an attempt to curb the spread of the virus. Over a billion students were directly affected by this globally. This decision was largely based on evidence that school closures could decrease transmission during influenza outbreaks (Jackson et al., 2014). Studies suggest that such measures also decreased transmission during COVID-19 or at least helped to flatten the curve. To uphold the right to education, teachers at primary, secondary and tertiary teaching facilities had to rapidly transition from in-person to online teaching. Despite their efforts, the quality of education was inevitably compromised; studies and exams were delayed, and students faced severe limitations in social interactions, which is an integral part of their education. Moreover, not all institutions globally had the same capacity to organise online education, and neither did all students have equal access to teaching materials. Approximately 463 million children were unable to engage in digital or broadcast learning during the widespread school closures. Vegas (2020) stated that roughly 65% of LMICs and less than 25% of low-income countries were able to set up online education and/or broadcast educational material. However, only 36% of residents of LMICs have access to the internet, making it challenging for students to follow online education. Even when internet access is available, it must be strong and reliable enough for effective learning. This issue is not confined to LMICs; in high-income countries, such as the Netherlands, less than 1% of children from poor families had access to online education due to insufficient internet access or devices (Save the Children Netherlands, 2020).

School closures not only impact students, teachers and families but have far-reaching economic and societal consequences. As parents are further confined to taking up educational activities for their children, they may not be able to work. The responsibility of facilitating these activities often falls on women, exacerbating existing gender inequalities. In sum, the right to education, despite the efforts of teaching institutions globally, was significantly compromised.

In relation to gender: the COVID-19 pandemic, especially the lockdown restrictions, exacerbated violence against women who were already in abusive situations and increased the number of women finding themselves in such circumstances. In an interview in the *Lancet*, Natalia Kanem, Executive Director of the UN Population Fund, stated that

> gender-based violence has distinguished the pandemic because of the lack of movement and people being trapped in abusive situations. The hotlines, the shelters, the counselling that is required has been increasing dramatically. It has happened in developed and developing countries.
>
> *(Cousins, 2020, p. 302)*

Furthermore, millions of women lost access to contraceptives due to the public health system being overwhelmed by COVID-19 and the mobility restrictions making it difficult to obtain contraceptives. UNFPA predicted there could be up to 7 million unintended pregnancies worldwide as a result of the crisis, potentially leading to thousands of deaths from unsafe abortions and complicated births due to inadequate access to emergency care (Cousins, 2020). For more information on reproductive rights and the rights of women, see Chapter 5 of this book.

In relation to the health care system: three key points related to health care systems merit discussion. First, health workers faced significant human rights dilemmas, undertaking immense efforts and assuming substantial risks. Second, access to care emerged as a critical issue. Third, the fundamental nature of our health system requires examination. During the COVID-19 outbreak, especially at the peak of the first wave, ICUs were overwhelmed, and practitioners grappled with tough ethical decisions about whom to treat. Should care be provided to all individuals, regardless of age or potential for recovery, or should the focus be on the young and those with higher chances of recovery? Furthermore, should physical contact between people in institutional care and their loved ones be restricted? Health systems and the health workforce were confronted with these challenging questions.

A recent study noted a potential association of COVID-19 related mortality with health care resource availability. Specifically, individuals experience more severe health outcomes from COVID-19 in areas where health care resources are less accessible and available. In such circumstances, certain communities – such as those with lower incomes, those living in remote areas or marginalised groups – are likely to encounter significant challenges in accessing the health care they needed. Furthermore, when vaccines became available, ethical questions arise as to who will receive them. According to the right to health, health care goods, facilities and services should be available in sufficient quantity, accessible to everyone without discrimination, respectful of medical ethics and culturally appropriate and scientifically and medically appropriate and of good quality.

COVID-19 placed immense pressure on public health systems, adversely affecting individuals who required routine medical care. The pandemic led to significant disruptions in the early detection and treatment of serious illnesses. For example, in the US, newly diagnosed cancer cases dropped by almost 40%, and cancer referrals in the UK dropped by 75% (Kaufman et al., 2020). In the Netherlands, over a couple of months the number of breast cancer and colon cancer diagnoses dropped by 2,000 and 1,000 cases, respectively, becoming significantly lower than the expected number of cases (Dinmohamed et al., 2020). Additionally, the WHO reports in the 2021 Malaria and TB reports that approximately 47,000 additional Malaria deaths and 100,000 additional TB deaths were recorded. National immunisation programs faced severe setbacks during the pandemic, struggling to recover, while vaccine hesitancy grew, partly due to the government's focus on COVID-19 vaccination. Access to antenatal care services plummeted worldwide, and mental health problems surged. Last, the surge in COVID-19 cases, coupled with difficult decision-making and the overall strain on health care systems, significantly impacted health care workers. They faced considerable risks, including contracting the virus in the course of their duties, enduring long working hours and experiencing psychological distress and fatigue (WHO, 2020).

The final point in relation to the health system is a more critical one. The IHR and the Siracusa principles indeed allow for rights infringements, such as during COVID-19 outbreaks. But, simultaneously, they mandate governments to be prepared for pandemics. It can be seriously questioned whether executives indeed prepared their countries for such events. Horton (2020), in *The COVID-19 Catastrophe,* demonstrates that there was ample evidence available that supported investments in pandemic preparedness. However, the global community did not do so. Health systems globally did not, by and large, have enough protective equipment at hand. Health institutions and networks did not have internalised protocols to deal with such outbreaks at hand and national governments hardly have done simulation exercises to prepare for such outbreaks.

The current health system's emphasis on treatment rather than prevention highlights a significant shortcoming. We prioritise care and cure over preventive measures, resulting in a population of "career patients". This approach becomes especially problematic in pandemics like COVID-19, where co-morbidities greatly increase the risk of severe symptoms, while good nutritional status and overall health serve as protective factors. The medical focus of our health system became apparent during the initial outbreak response, with efforts concentrated on scaling-up ICU capacities, rather than expanding access to preventive measures or protections for frontline workers. These frontline health workers, the doctors and nurses who represent the care system, were lauded as the heroes of the pandemic. In contrast, public health institutions and providers, who were crucial in advising on public health measures, testing and contact tracing, faced substantial criticism. Ironically, these were the same entities that had previously advocated for increased investment in pandemic preparedness.

Vaccine inequality: human rights are universal, however, in practice this seems like an illusion when looking at access to COVID-19 vaccination. As of 1 October 2021, the wealthiest nations, as designated by the World Bank, boasted a per-capita vaccination rate of 125.3 vaccinations per 100 individuals. This figure stands nearly three times higher than the rate observed in lower-middle-income countries – which was 45.3 per 100 – and a staggering 30 times higher than in lower-income countries, where it stood at 4.2 per 100 (World Bank). Also within countries inequities persisted, where generally those with low wealth or educational status or coming from ethnic minorities had lower access.

To improve vaccine equality, COVAX, short for COVID-19 Vaccines Global Access, was launched in April 2020. It aimed to ensure equitable access to COVID-19 vaccines worldwide, particularly for lower-income countries that might otherwise struggle to afford or secure access to vaccines. However, from the start, COVAX faced obstacles including vaccine nationalism in affluent nations, commercial concerns and, notably, a discrepancy between the timing of funding availability and the demand for vaccines (Usher, 2023). The competition between countries that were supposed to support COVAX but instead prioritised their own vaccine supplies, highlighted a troubling disparity in the interpretation of human rights. It became evident that some governments viewed human rights as "citizen rights" rather than "universal rights". This perspective suggested that the right of their own citizens to access vaccines was deemed more important than ensuring equitable vaccine distribution for all people globally.

The principle of equality between diseases: while avoiding a detailed discussion on the costs associated with COVID-19 and the quality-adjusted life years gained, a pressing question remains: is it equitable to allocate billions of dollars to COVID-19 while spending only a fraction of that amount on diseases like tuberculosis, which claims over a million lives annually (Wingfield et al., 2020)? Moreover, what about the many other diseases that also require attention? Health economists often assess the cost-effectiveness of health interventions, evaluating how much is spent or saved per quality-adjusted life year gained. Researchers have long identified numerous cost-effective and cost-saving interventions that can prevent major causes of death and disability, such as tuberculosis and common maternal and child health issues. Despite this, many of these interventions remain underutilised and are simply not implemented. In contrast, there has been considerable debate over whether the measures implemented to control COVID-19 were truly cost-effective. Assessing this is complex for several reasons. First, the benefits of the measures are difficult to determine – as they should prevent COVID-19 cases and simultaneously reduce pressure on care providers to perform "routine care". Second, the negative side effects of the measures are very uncertain (e.g., increase in mental health problems, long-term effects of food insecurity). Finally, evaluating indirect costs is difficult, and whether the measures exacerbated the economic crisis or contributed to its resolution remains unclear.

COVID-19 and Decision-making

The aforementioned human rights infringements during the COVID-19 pandemic could easily have been mistaken for a battering of COVID-19 responses. This is by no means my intention. It serves to demonstrate some of the trade-offs that needed to be made. Remember, doing absolutely nothing would most likely have been a much greater negligence of human rights. The aforementioned points, however, do show how difficult it is to make decisions during COVID-19. In terms of moral frameworks, a deontological approach may lead to inaction as moral principles are conflicting; a consequentialist approach is difficult as the effects of measures are uncertain. Decisions have to be made that are proportional, and we should ensure that the treatment is not worse than the illness.

Two critiques on the decision-making processes merit discussion, including i) that decision-making was not timely because of the decision-making paradigm based on "evidence-based medicine"; ii) that decision-making was largely authoritarian which does not match local realities. Another critique on decision-making – the lack of pandemic preparedness – has been covered earlier in this chapter.

> The response of governments to COVID-19 represents the greatest political failure of Western democracies since the Second World War. A government's first responsibility is its duty of care to citizens. Early government inaction led to the avoidable deaths of thousands of those citizens. The failures were legion.
>
> *(Horton, 2020, p. 84)*

In his book on the COVID-19 catastrophe, Horton emphasises that states made decisions too late, despite scientific evidence and evidence from affected states. Country after country seemed to make the same mistakes and implement measures too late, with limited vision and with poor communication. Why did countries like the Netherlands, the UK and the US not learn from the catastrophe in countries like Italy to implement measures sooner? Similarly, Greenhalgh (2020) states that the UK government and their advisors have relied too much on the decision-making paradigm of evidence-based medicine: an approach that is based on evidence from RCTs and systemic reviews to establish generalisable cause and effects relations, to make decisions. Without doubt, evidence-based medicine is crucial to identify safe and effective treatments – also for COVID-19. However, in our complex societies "such precise quantification of cause-effect relationships is both impossible (because such relationships are not constant and cannot be meaningfully isolated) and unnecessary (because what matters is what emerges in a particular unique situation)" (ibidem, p. 2).

During the COVID-19 outbreak, the multitude of interacting factors were highly unpredictable; a more prudent approach to decision-making would involve naturalistic methods, where scientists observe and even participate in real-world phenomena, as in anthropological fieldwork and rapid-cycle evaluation. That is, collecting data in a systematic but pragmatic way and feeding it back in a timely way to inform ongoing improvement. To make this concrete, Greenhalgh argues that there was ample evidence from, for example, modelling studies, narrative reviews and experiences of past pandemics that could have been used to develop policy. Neglecting such evidence, which may not meet the standards of evidence-based medicine and at times may even be heavily contested (e.g., wearing face-masks), would be irrational and lead to an unacceptable standstill in decision-making. Concurrently, it would be irrational to use this evidence naively. Decision-makers should accept their "bounded rationality" as there is no agreement of relevant evidence and relevant values and rather engage with a policy of learning (see e.g., Hisschemöller & Hoppe, 1995; Simon, 1982) in which policy is formulated based on available evidence and constantly adjusted to progressive insights from rapid cycles of reflection. The paradigm for evidence-based medicine is ill-suited for public health practice.

"We need to fight COVID-19!" Loewenson and colleagues (2020) argue that such a warlike rhetoric practised during the COVID-19 pandemic in itself undermines human rights (see also Marya & Patel, 2021). They argue that the decisions during the pandemic were "made and enforced in an overcentralised, non-transparent, top-down manner". These were also dubbed a "biosecurity-focused, authoritarian and sometimes militarised approaches to public health", in which a selective group of high-ranked government officials and a selective group of academics make decisions. This has led to decisions being made from a largely biomedical perspective and enforced in an overcentralised manner. Proponents will argue that this will speed up decision-making and create clarity. However, these methods often involve military coercion and abuse in communities, even while evidence shows the long-term harm to public health and human rights. The militant rhetoric and the often one-size-fits-all measures that we take to fight COVID-19 may not do justice to the diverse contexts in which people are situated. It is not difficult to imagine how a one-size-fits-all policy may have very different consequences for different communities and may require different implementation models. For example, overcrowded poor townships of Cape Town are totally different than the more affluent neighbourhoods of the same city. An alternative approach should be comprehensive, emphasise social determinants, be participatory and be rights based. This would imply an approach that decentralises policy-making, acknowledging the specific needs and capacities of local communities. Participatory approaches will contribute to policies that are i) better informed, as different perspectives are included; ii) more supported, because those affected are involved in their making and iii) more legitimate, as people have the right to be involved in policy-making that affects them. In such a participatory process it is crucial that actors from science and society try to understand and engage with one another's' perspective to develop a course of action. The question may arise that such processes may lead to unnecessary delays in decision-making. It therefore remains crucial to commit to rapid cycles of action and reflection. In Textbox 11.3 on the outbreak management teams (OMTs) we raised the question whether all relevant perspectives are included in the OMTs. In Textbox 11.4, another thought experiment is presented that will stimulate thinking about how COVID-19 infection and measures to prevent this affect people differently.

Both critiques on the decision-making process provide relevant insights to respond to a public health crisis while taking human rights into account. On such a complex issue as COVID-19, where evidence is limited, contested and at times conflicting, decision-making – and decision-makers – have to accept that our "rationality is bounded" (cf. Simon, 1982). A policy of learning with actors from science and society is required, in which rapid cycles of action and reflection should be used to formulate, implement, observe and adapt policy. This is in accordance with the argument made by Hamelink in Chapter 3 of this book "in the resolution of moral choices in real-life situations we may need to move to a contextual ethics: in the form of a regular and systematic dialogue".

Textbox 11.3
Composition of Outbreak Management Teams

In the event of a nation-wide outbreak of infectious disease, taskforces can be set up in a country to monitor and control the outbreak. For example, in the Netherlands, the Centre for the Control of Infectious Disease (RIVM-CIb) played a coordinating role in controlling the COVID-19 outbreak. Further, the RIVM established an Outbreak Management Team (OMT) that *advised* the government, as the government was responsible for decision-making.

Question for Discussion

- In your country, check whether such an OMT was established and explore the list of experts consulted. Do you think the participants were diverse? What other expertise would you want to see in the OMT (if any)?

Textbox 11.4
Mandatory Vaccination?

It is argued that if a lockdown is compatible with human rights – limiting the freedom of movement – so is compulsory vaccination. However, this is simply by law not allowed; it is actually assault when given without consent. In the Covenant on Civil and Political Rights it is stated that certain rights cannot be derogated: including the right not to be subject of inhuman or degrading treatment. Mandatory vaccination conflicts with the autonomy of individuals and the integrity of their bodies. Compulsory interference with a person's bodily integrity is not something that a democratic society will tolerate without detailed regulations and specialist tribunals in place. Lack of mental capacity coupled with risk to health of the individual and to the public is the only justification we have for such a draconian measure. The more important discussion will be on "who gets the vaccine", for example, groups at risk for severe disease progression or groups critical in the chain of transmission and "to what extent do we limit people's freedom who have not been vaccinated"? For example, will health care workers that are not vaccinated be able to work with the elderly? Or will I, when I am not vaccinated, be allowed to visit a music concert? I believe that the actual human rights discussion will be on these issues. Here we need to be very cautious and pragmatic. Cautious as we want to prevent people who want to participate in society feeling forced to be vaccinated and to prevent unnecessary discrimination. Pragmatic, as we have as of yet limited availability of vaccines and resources to provide everybody the opportunity quickly to get vaccinated.

Question for Discussion

- Argue why we should or should not limit the freedom of individuals not vaccinated against COVID-19 when a vaccine is available publicly and COVID-19 transmission still occurs.

Concluding Remarks

Public health emergencies, such as infectious disease outbreaks, may require limiting the rights of individuals to protect the public. In this chapter we have discussed the International Health Regulations that provide a framework for responding to such outbreaks. This and other legal frameworks provide guidance on measures and decision-making that take into account the rights of individuals and the public. The COVID-19 example showed that such an outbreak and its measures have far-reaching (human rights) implications. Decision-making in such events is extremely difficult; a deontological approach may lead to inaction as moral principles are conflicting; a consequentialist approach is difficult as the effects of measures are uncertain. Large-scale public health emergencies, such as pandemics, require action that is proportional and fitted to the context where they are made.

The COVID-19 pandemic illustrates a story of state failure to prioritise human rights. Future pandemics should rigorously monitor human rights, covering not only the right to health but also political, civil, economic, social and cultural rights. Furthermore, equity must be ensured both between and within countries. This can be achieved by making health technology and products accessible globally and tailoring approaches within countries to address the needs of all individuals.

Questions for Discussion

- Discuss whether the legal framework of the IHR sufficiently safeguards the rights of the individual.
- Discuss from a human rights perspective whether the measures implemented to prevent COVID-19 treatment did more harm than good. Was the "treatment" of COVID-19 worse than the illness?
- Discuss what (other) human rights infringements you observed during the COVID-19 pandemic.
- Discuss what human rights infringements you experienced during the outbreak, and whether you consider these fair.
- Discuss whether an authoritarian approach to deal with pandemics is appropriate.
- Discuss whether you think the new regulations and treaties, which are formulated to provide judicial support for measures to address Public Health Emergencies of International Concern, in the long run disproportionally affect human rights.

References

Ahmed, F., Ahmed, N., Pissarides, C., & Stiglitz, J. (2020). Why inequality could spread COVID-19. *The Lancet Public Health*, 2667(20), 30085.

Angeli, F., & Montefusco, A. (2020). Sensemaking and learning during the COVID-19 pandemic: A complex adaptive systems perspective on policy decision-making. *World Development*, *136*, 105106.

Anthem, P. (2020). *Risk of hunger pandemic as coronavirus set to almost double acute hunger by end of 2020* (Vol. 16). World Food Programme Insight. https://www.wfp.org/stories/risk-hunger-pandemic-coronavirus-set-almost-double-acute-hunger-end-2020

Arceo-Gomez, E. O., Campos-Vazquez, R. M., Esquivel, G., Alcaraz, E., Martinez, L. A., & Lopez, N. G. (2022). The income gradient in COVID-19 mortality and hospitalisation: An observational study with social security administrative records in Mexico. *The Lancet Regional Health-Americas*, 6.

Barro, R. J., Ursúa, J. F., & Weng, J. (2020). *The coronavirus and the great influenza pandemic: Lessons from the "Spanish flu" for the coronavirus's potential effects on mortality and economic activity* (No. w26866). National Bureau of Economic Research.

Bennett, B., & Carney, T. (2017). Public health emergencies of international concern: Global, regional, and local responses to risk. *Medical Law Review*, 25(2), 223–239.

CDC. (2022). *COVID-19 hospitalization and death by race/ethnicity*. https://archive.cdc.gov/www_cdc_gov/coronavirus/2019-ncov/COVID-data/investigations-discovery/hospitalization-death-by-race-ethnicity.html

Chan, M. (2007). Message from the director general. In *A safer future: Global public health security in the 21st century* (pp. vi–vii). World Health Organization.

Chorus, C., Sandorf, E. D., & Mouter, N. (2020). Diabolical dilemmas of COVID-19: An empirical study into Dutch society's trade-offs between health impacts and other effects of the lockdown. *PLoS One*, 15(9), e0238683.

Christensen, J. G., & Mortensen, P. B. (2024). Coping with the unforeseen: Bounded rationality and bureaucratic responses to the COVID-19 crisis. *Journal of Public Policy*, 44(1), 24–43.

Cousins, S. (2020). COVID-19 has "devastating" effect on women and girls. *The Lancet*, 396(10247), 301–302.

Davies, S. E., & Bennett, B. (2016). A gendered human rights analysis of Ebola and Zika: Locating gender in global health emergencies. *International Affairs*, 92(5), 1041–1060.

Dinmohamed, A. G., Cellamare, M., Visser, O., de Munck, L., Elferink, M. A., Westenend, P. J., Wesseling, J., Broeders, M. J. M., Kuipers, E. J., Merkx, M. A. W., Nagtegaal, I. D., & Siesling, S. (2020). The impact of the temporary suspension of national cancer screening programmes due to the COVID-19 epidemic on the diagnosis of breast and colorectal cancer in the Netherlands. *Journal of Hematology & Oncology*, 13, 1–4.

Gelfand, M. J., Jackson, J. C., Pan, X., Nau, D., Pieper, D., Denison, E., Dagher, M., Van Lange, P. A. M., Chiu, C.-Y., & Wang, M. (2021). The relationship between cultural tightness–looseness and COVID-19 cases and deaths: A global analysis. *The Lancet Planetary Health*, 5(3), e135–e144.

Gostin, L. O., Friedman, E. A., Hossain, S., Mukherjee, J., Zia-Zarifi, S., Clinton, C., Rugege, U., Buss, P., Were, M., & Dhai, A. (2023). Human rights and the COVID-19 pandemic: A retrospective and prospective analysis. *The Lancet*, 401(10371), 154–168.

Greenhalgh, T. (2020). Will COVID-19 be evidence-based medicine's nemesis? *PLOS Medicine*, 17(6), e1003266.

Hankivsky, O., & Kapilashrami, A. (2020). *Beyond sex and gender analysis: An intersectional view of the COVID-19 pandemic outbreak and response*. Gender and Women's Health Unit, School of Population and Health Equity.

Heymann, D. L., Prentice, T., & Reinders, L. T. (2007). *The world health report 2007: A safer future: Global public health security in the 21st century*. World Health Organization.

Hisschemöller, M., & Hoppe, R. (1995). Coping with intractable controversies: The case for problem structuring in policy design and analysis. *Knowledge and Policy*, 8(4), 40–60.

Horton, R. (2020). *The COVID-19 catastrophe: What's gone wrong and how to stop it happening again*. Polity Press.

Jackson, C., Mangtani, P., Hawker, J., Olowokure, B., & Vynnycky, E. (2014). The effects of school closures on influenza outbreaks and pandemics: Systematic review of simulation studies. *PLOS One*, 9(5), e97297.

Kaufman, H. W., Chen, Z., Niles, J., & Fesko, Y. (2020). Changes in the number of US patients with newly identified cancer before and during the coronavirus disease 2019 (COVID-19) pandemic. *JAMA Network Open*, 3(8), e2017267.

The Lancet Global Health. (2020). Decolonising COVID-19. *The Lancet Global Health*, 8(5), e612.

Landry, M. D., Geddes, L., Moseman, A. P., Lefler, J. P., Raman, S. R., & van Wijchen, J. (2020). Early reflection on the global impact of COVID19, and implications for physiotherapy. *Physiotherapy*, 107, A1–A3.

Levin, A. T., Owusu-Boaitey, N., Pugh, S., Fosdick, B. K., Zwi, A. B., Malani, A., Soman, S., Besançon, L., Kashnitsky, I., Ganesh, S., McLaughlin, A., Song, G., Uhm, R., Herrera-Esposito, D., de Los Campos, G., Antonio, A. C. P. P., Tadese, E. B., & Meyerowitz-Katz, G. (2022). Assessing the burden of COVID-19 in developing countries: Systematic review, meta-analysis and public policy implications. *BMJ Global Health*, 7(5), e008477.

Loewenson, R., Accoe, K., Bajpai, N., Buse, K., Abi Deivanayagam, T., London, L., Méndez, C. A., Mirzoev, T., Nelson, E., Parray, A. A., & Probandari, A. (2020). Reclaiming comprehensive public health. *BMJ Global Health*, 5(9), e003886.

Mander, H. (2020). State's measures to fight coronavirus are stripping the poor of dignity and hope. *The Indian Express*. https://indianexpress.com/article/opinion/columns/coronavirus-covid-19-lockdown-poor-6333452/

Marya, R., & Patel, R. (2021). *Inflamed: Deep medicine and the anatomy of injustice*. Penguin.

McKeever, V. (2020). The coronavirus is expected to have cost 400 million jobs in the second quarter, UN labor agency estimates. *CNBC*. https://www.cnbc.com/2020/06/30/coronavirus-expected-to-cost-400-million-jobs-in-the-second-quarter.html

Mullen, L., Potter, C., Gostin, L. O., Cicero, A., & Nuzzo, J. B. (2020). An analysis of international health regulations emergency committees and public health emergency of international concern designations. *BMJ Global Health*, 5(6), e002502.

Murphy, T. (2013). *Health and human rights*. Hart Publishing Ltd.

OECD. (2020, June 11). *G20 GDP growth – first quarter of 2020*. OECD. Retrieved September 6, 2020.

Oshitani, H., Kamigaki, T., & Suzuki, A. (2008). Major issues and challenges of influenza pandemic preparedness in developing countries. *Emerging Infectious Diseases, 14*(6), 875–880.

Phua, K. L. (2015). Meeting the challenge of Ebola virus disease in a holistic manner by taking into account socioeconomic and cultural factors: The experience of West Africa. *Infectious Diseases: Research and Treatment, 8*, IDRT-S31568.

Rajkumar, R. P. (2023). Cultural values and changes in happiness in 78 countries during the COVID-19 pandemic: An analysis of data from the world happiness reports. *Frontiers in Psychology, 14*, 1090340.

Rittel, H. W., & Webber, M. M. (1973). Dilemmas in a general theory of planning. *Policy Sciences, 4*(2), 155–169.

Save the Children Netherlands. (2020). *COVID-19: Kinderen uit arme gezinnen het meest getroffen door pandemie*. https://www.savethechildren.nl/actueel/nieuws/2020/COVID-19-kinderen-uit-arme-gezinnen-het-meest-get

Simon, H. A. (1982). *Models of bounded rationality*. MIT Press.

Smith, J. A., & Judd, J. (2020). COVID-19: Vulnerability and the power of privilege in a pandemic. *Health Promotion Journal of Australia, 31*(2), 158.

Song, S., & Choi, Y. (2023). Differences in the COVID-19 pandemic response between South Korea and the United States: A comparative analysis of culture and policies. *Journal of Asian and African Studies, 58*(2), 196–213.

Stemple, L., Karegeya, P., & Gruskin, S. (2016). Human rights, gender, and infectious disease: From HIV/AIDS to Ebola. *Human Rights Quarterly, 38*(4), 993–1021.

UN. (1984). *Siracusa principles on the limitation and derogation of provisions in the ICCPR* (UN Doc. No. E/CN). UN.

Upshur, R. E. (2002). Principles for the justification of public health intervention. *Canadian Journal of Public Health, 93*(2), 101–103.

Usher, A. D. (2023). COVAX: The unspent billions. *The Lancet, 402*(10408), 1119–1122.

van Vliet, J. A., Haringhuizen, G. B., Timen, A., & Bijkerk, P. (2009). Changes in the duty of notification of infectious diseases via the Dutch public health act. *Nederlands Tijdschrift voor Geneeskunde, 153*, B79.

Vegas, E. (2020). *School closures, government responses, and learning inequality around the world during COVID-19*. Brookings Institution.

Vieira, C. M., Franco, O. H., Restrepo, C. G., & Abel, T. (2020). COVID-19: The forgotten priorities of the pandemic. *Maturitas, 136*, 38–41.

Wenham, C., Smith, J., & Morgan, R. (2020). COVID-19: The gendered impacts of the outbreak. *The Lancet, 395*(10227), 846–848.

WHO. (2008). *International health regulations (2005)*. World Health Organization.

WHO. (2020). *Coronavirus disease (COVID-19) outbreak: Rights, roles and responsibilities of health workers, including key considerations for occupational safety and health: Interim guidance*, 19 March 2020.

Wingfield, T., Cuevas, L. E., MacPherson, P., Millington, K. A., & Squire, S. B. (2020). Tackling two pandemics: A plea on world tuberculosis day. *The Lancet Respiratory Medicine, 8*(6), 536.

Yerkes, M. A., André, S. C. H., Besamusca, J. W., Hummel, B., Remery, C., van der Zwan, R., Kruyen, P. M., Beckers, D. G. J., & Geurts, S. A. E. (2020). *COGIS-NL: COVID Gender (In)equality Survey Netherlands: Second policy brief: Results from June*. https://repository.ubn.ru.nl/handle/2066/228387

Zidar, A. (2015). WHO international health regulations and human rights: From allusions to inclusion. *The International Journal of Human Rights, 19*(4), 505–526.

For Further Reading

Horton, R. (2020). *The COVID-19 catastrophe: What's gone wrong and how to stop it happening again*. Polity Press.

Loewenson, R., Accoe, K., Bajpai, N., Buse, K., Abi Deivanayagam, T., London, L., Méndez, C. A., Mirzoev, T., Nelson, E., Parray, A. A., & Probandari, A. (2020). Reclaiming comprehensive public health. *BMJ Global Health*, *5*(9), e003886.

Marya, R., & Patel, R. (2021). *Inflamed: Deep medicine and the anatomy of injustice*. Penguin.

Zidar, A. (2015). WHO international health regulations and human rights: From allusions to inclusion. *The International Journal of Human Rights*, *19*(4), 505–526.

CHAPTER 12

Technology and the Right to Health

Cees J. Hamelink and Dirk R. Essink

Introduction

The right of access to advances in technology is provided in Article 27.1. of the Universal Declaration of Human Rights where it is stated that "Everyone has the right to . . . share in scientific advancement and its benefits". This right is inspired by the basic moral principle of equality and the notion that science and technology belong to the common heritage of humankind. This chapter will discuss how the right provided in Article 27 applies to the right to health. Since crucial choices will have to be made in relation to advances in medical technology, we will also look into responsible ways of planning future choices. We propose a human rights-based assessment of stories about possible futures.

Learning Objectives
After studying this chapter you will be able to:

- Understand the complex relationship between advances in medical technology and the protection of the right to health
- Discuss the need for a human rights assessment of technology choices
- Understand the importance of accounting for technology choices
- Better manage decision-making on future applications of medical technology

Human Rights and Technology
Up until 1968 there was no serious debate in the international community about the relation between scientific and technological development and the protection of human rights. At the Teheran International Conference on Human Rights (1968), the following statement was adopted: "while recent scientific discoveries and technological advances have opened vast prospects for economic, social and cultural progress, such developments may nevertheless endanger rights and freedoms of individuals and will require continuing attention". The Conference recommended in Resolution XI "that the

DOI: 10.4324/9781003408765-16

organizations of the United Nations family should undertake a study of the problems with respect to human rights arising from developments in science and technology". In the years 1971–1976, a series of reports was produced dealing with the problems of privacy protection, use of observation satellites, automation, procedures of prenatal diagnosis, introduction of chemicals into food production, deterioration of the environment and the destructive power of modern weapons systems.

On November 10, 1975 the General Assembly resolved to adopt the Declaration on the Use of Scientific and Technological Progress in the Interests of Peace and for the Benefit of Mankind (UNGA res. 3384).

Among the key principles of the declaration are:

- International cooperation to ensure that the results of science and technology developments are used to strengthen international peace and security; to promote economic and social development and to realise human rights and freedoms.
- Measures to ensure that science and technology developments satisfy the material and the spiritual needs of all people.
- Measures to extend the benefits of science and technology developments to all strata of the population and to protect them against all possible harmful effects.
- Measures to ensure that the use of science and technology developments promotes the realisation of human rights.
- Measures to prevent the use of science and technology development to the detriment of human rights.

In September 1975, a meeting of experts took place in Geneva which recommended the establishment of an international machinery for the assessment of new technologies from the point of view of human rights. This form of technology assessment would include the evaluation of possible side-effects and long-range effects of technological innovations and would weigh the advantages of such innovations against disadvantages. The General Assembly did not act upon this recommendation.

Technology and the Protection Against Harmful Effects

The UN Commission on Human Rights and the General Assembly have over past decades on several occasions drawn attention to the observation that people not only derive benefits from the use of advances in technology but can also be negatively affected by them. There is an awareness of the potentially harmful effects of new technologies on the physical and mental integrity of people (through new forms of personal and bodily tests), on the privacy and confidentiality of their homes and correspondence (through new forms of surveillance), on the deterioration of people's working environments (through automation techniques) and on the natural environment (as a result of the dumping of electric and electronic waste).

Technology and Decision-making

The idea of human rights has to extend to the social institutions (the institutional arrangements) that would facilitate the realisation of fundamental standards. Human rights cannot be realised without involving citizens in the decision-making processes about the spheres in which freedom and equality are to be achieved. This moves the democratic process beyond the political sphere and extends the requirement of participatory institutional arrangements to other social domains. The human right to democratic participation claims that technology choices also should be subject to democratic control. This is particularly important in light of the fact that current political processes tend to delegate important areas of social life to private rather than to public control and accountability. Increasingly large volumes of social activity are withdrawn from public accountability, from democratic control and from the participation of citizens in decision-making. Technology has rarely ever been invented, developed and applied under the guidance of normative, moral principles. Engineerability was and is – often in combination with commercial or military interest – the essential driving force.

Dependence Versus Autonomy

As a result of technological development, there is an ever increasing number of tools and instruments that are ill-understood by their human users. Throughout our daily routines we use pieces of electrical and electronic equipment (varying from ATMs, cell phones, cars and self-check-in systems at airports to microwave ovens) that function on the basis of complex hardware and software technologies which few of us master. As a matter of fact, increasingly today's advanced technologies exceed the knowledge and skills of even well-trained specialists. Whereas people could fairly easily learn how to repair their bikes, with cars loaded with digital gadgets there is almost complete dependence upon the expert who is increasingly dependent upon computerised data-systems that "think and decide" for the expert. Advancements in artificial intelligence (AI), nanotechnology, biotechnology and robotics reinforce a process of knowledge "extensification" that places the processing and understanding of knowledge increasingly under the control of intelligent tools and instruments. In this process, human beings may begin to lose their autonomy over the acquisition of knowledge and become dependent upon digital copies and electronic searches.

Vulnerability Versus Integrity

With the increasing dependence upon advanced technology we become more vulnerable to its malfunctioning as a result of systemic flaws or deliberate misuse. An inescapable part of living in modernity is that – as Ulrich Beck (1992) has proposed – we live in a "risk society". Also the deployment of advanced systems in medical technology implies vulnerability to malfunctioning of the technological infrastructure due to software failures, managerial incompetence, increasing complexity of technical systems and even the deliberate destruction of computer systems.

Choices

The space within which human choices are made is limited. When it comes to such essential choices as the times of birth and death, the type of gender and race or the quality of health and intelligence, there is little freedom to choose. Yet, there remain many situations where we can take different routes and can say "Yes" or "No".

As we argued earlier in the chapter on the human rights methods of ethics, implicit in the realisation that we make choices – and often choices that critically affect others – is the responsibility to account for them! Therefore, we may be asked to defend our moral choices and expose the mental map that guides our choices to public scrutiny. This holds equally for the designers, developers and manufacturers of modern technology as for the policy-makers and regulators and also the corporate and private users. From a human rights perspective, this means that we question how inventions, developments and innovations in technology affect the respect for human dignity, autonomy, equality and security. There may hardly ever be the guarantee that a given choice is optimal, but at least choices can be accounted for beyond the common arguments of profit, greed or selfish interest. In the spirit of a discursive process all the stakeholders should design visions for possible futures that either promote or violate the basic human rights values.

Limits to the Access of Technological Advances

The increase in costs for technology is arguably the main driver for increasing costs for health care. And the increasing costs for care are the main barrier to keeping health care accessible for all. For example, wider availability of technologies such as magnetic resonance imaging (MRI), computed tomography (CT), coronary artery bypass grafting, angioplasty, cardiac and neonatal intensive care units, positron emission tomography (PET) and radiation oncology facilities correlates with higher per capita utilisation and greater spending on these services. Also, it is hard to determine whether access to technologies is always medically warranted. Unlimited access to these technologies is in most health care systems unattainable, and an illusion is most of the Global South. To ensure access to the benefits of technology, limited access may be needed.

Human Rights Assessment

In 1975 the meeting of experts in Geneva that was referred to earlier recommended to the UN General Assembly the establishment of an international machinery for the assessment of new technologies from the point of view of human rights. Almost a half century later, the recommendation still makes eminent sense.

Procedure

Following human rights standards, the assessment process would have to be organised through democratic arrangements. This implies the broadest possible participation of all people in processes of public decision-making that affect their well-being. Therefore, forms of participatory democracy have to be designed for policymaking in the sphere of the production, development and dissemination of medical technology. This conflicts with the observation that there is presently a widening gap between the domains of technological development and political decision-making (Winner, 1993). The development of biotechnology provides a good illustration. Scientists and investors cooperate to produce artificial tissue, blood vessels and organs such as hearts and livers. Developments in the field of "regenerative" medicine may start a process of renovating human beings. It is expected that the bio industry will soon bring a veritable "body shop" with human spare parts on the market. Irrespective of its possible advantages versus disadvantages, the whole process evolves outside any form of social control. Social concerns and anxieties about developments in genetic technology do not seem to have an impact on the real decisions in this domain. These decisions have already been taken because the question of whether certain developments were socially desirable was never posed. The future course is determined outside the political domain as choices of technology and its application are not made by the political system. Investment decisions count more than considerations of common welfare. However, if democracy represents the notion that all people should participate in those decisions that shape their future welfare, such social forces as medical technologies cannot just be left to the interests and stakes of commercial parties on the market-place.

Advanced medical treatment methods may have serious implications for the rights and freedoms of all those affected by them. Artificial methods of reproduction such as in-vitro fertilisation (IVF), egg donation, embryo donation and surrogacy relate to the human right to found a family, the protection of privacy, freedom of scientific research and the right of children to obtain information about their parents. The screening for hereditary disorders or diagnosing metabolic disorders implies human rights aspects such as maximising the right to health and the right to life. But there are also risks of threats to human dignity, to privacy rights, to political rights and to the freedom of movement. Much-contested issues are the genetic passport and the option of compulsory medical examination. Medical genetics implies risks for personal privacy, breaches of confidentiality and threats to the right to physical integrity. A crucial human rights aspect is "informed consent". The person to be examined should consent to the intervention on the basis of sufficient knowledge and understanding of all aspects and implications of the examinations. The "informed consent" rule can only be omitted in exceptional and carefully defined circumstances. Governments have considerable discretionary power of balance in public and private interests. However, this has to be a careful process in which the question of whether the desired result can be achieved under less restrictive measures should always be considered. The rights to human dignity and physical integrity are at stake as well as the rights to work, housing, social security and participation in cultural life. Often in these situations the right to equality is under threat. It is of particular importance to question the importance of the non-discrimination standard in relation to measures (both in state–citizen vertical relations and citizen-to-citizen horizontal relations) that imply restrictions on the basis of health status.

Risks for human well-being also stem from advances in bio-technology as they enable genetic manipulation, laboratory synthesis of bacterial genomes or the re-creation of a lethal virus (polio virus or Spanish influenza virus). These advances may come with enormous benefits in medical treatments but may also be misused and threaten human security. "It remains unclear how civilization can ensure that it reaps the benefits of biotechnology while protecting itself from the worst misuse" (Nouri & Chyba, 2008, p. 451). As Nouri and Chyba argue, there are at present no adequate regulatory schemes to deal with the rapid and widespread advances in biotechnology (ibidem). From a human rights perspective, securing biological security is an urgent concern on the agenda of the right to health.

The Application of Artificial Intelligence (AI)

A special dimension of current technological developments is the design of AI and its application in so-called expert systems. AI research attempts to replicate human brain capacity in digital systems, and it tries to find forms of man/machine symbiosis that enlarge the problem-solving capacities of both human beings and machines. Present discussions focus on the possible effects of intelligent robotic systems on employment and the use of expert systems in health care. It is quite common to criticise or ridicule the pretentious forecasts of the AI community. It is indeed true that many excited claims by AI researchers have never materialised. Critics argue that the nature of human intelligence and the limits of machine thinking render it futile to reflect on future forms of new and intelligent life. However, this criticism is based on the flawed assumption that certain developments will not occur, because we presently hold them to be unrealistic. This is not a convincing argument against the possibility that what we currently perceive as fiction could be realised in the future. AI research raises moral issues that were not posed by other technologies. Let us assume that new types of human intelligence could be developed that would be superior to the capacities of the human species. The confrontation between the human being and the humanoid digital system (the "cyborg") creates a fundamentally new situation for moral philosophy. The cyborg presupposes a development by which digital electronics is deployed within the human body and human brainpower is linked to cybernetic systems. This would seem to belong to the realm of science fiction, and there is indeed no possibility to predict with any certainty which forms of digital life this leads us to. Because there are no indications that human beings will be held back by moral considerations in the search for the possibility of "virtual people", it is only reasonable to not discard the evolution of a new humanoid species that is more intelligent than human beings. This development would imply that, for the first time in their history, human beings have to cooperate with a different species. The relations between human beings and other species were never based on cooperation. Whatever feelings people may have for animals, they never cooperate with them. People have never negotiated with other species about coexistence. The cyborg would force humans to do so. In this confrontation, it may turn out that our moral rules are too human-centric. Many animals have suffered from this but could not negotiate with humans about a change of the moral canon. The new species could do just this and challenge the human being to design a morality that takes all sentient beings seriously. In many societies, solemn debates will take place about the morality of producing digital clones of human persons and the implied threats for human autonomy. In the end, the overriding factor is likely to be the question of whether there is a market for the intelligent cyborg. Current developments with the application of intelligent tools already have begun to erode human autonomy. This is the case when moral choice making is "outsourced" to applications of digital technology. Whenever digital technologies (or any other technologies for that matter) make decisions, the moral development of human beings will stop because they no longer learn from making moral mistakes. Privacy-enhancing technologies take away from the human actor the moral responsibility to protect his or her privacy. Advanced medical diagnostic systems shift moral responsibility from medical staff to computer software or at least reduce the autonomous space for moral choice by human operators.

A Normative Position

Throughout its evolutionary journey, the human species has always found flexible ways to adapt to changing environments. The history of human moral evolution has not ended. In the 21st century, the human species finds a new environment to adapt to: the ubiquitous robotic environment. In this environment, all essential infrastructures for societal life are transformed by a convergence technology that brings together informatics, telecommunications technology, robotics, biotechnology and AI. The exponential rate at which convergence technology develops leads us into an arena in which humanoid robots will become increasingly essential and could eventually take over many human tasks. This raises the most existential question of all: does the future need us? When we began to "automobilise" our environment, we adapted by creating rules, enforcement measures, training courses and driver's licenses. Without this framework, the mess in traffic would have even been bigger than it is today. The digitising of our environment is a much more encompassing project, and we seem to lack guidance for the moral choices we have to make on burning issues such as net neutrality, privacy protection, big data, surveillance, free speech, security, Facebook terrorism, technology divides and Twitter intimidation.

What should be the basic normative position? The human rights regime as our moral compass represents the search for a normative foundation. Human rights in robotic times address the core question of whether we can manage our societies – virtual and real – such as to make them caring, convivial, egalitarian and secure. It seems unlikely to me that we can achieve this if we leave the decisions about the future to the forces and interests of neo-liberal politics and capitalist economies. They are too much driven by the evils of selfishness, greed, injustice, lack of compassion and the need to dominate. A human rights-based future may require us to be intensely human by doing what we learned in our evolutionary past. We are good as social beings, we have cooperative skills, we form teams, we are empathic, we are co-creative and we are story-tellers. Many applications of advanced technologies will lead to complex moral issues and the need for ethical reflection. In modern times humans are challenged to make moral choices, to make them in uncertainty and to account for them.

Concluding Remarks

Humanity is confronted with great and rapid advances in forms of technology that have strong impacts on human physical and mental well-being. The most dramatic global risk is the possibility of global warfare in which computer technology, nanotechnology and biotechnology could play a major role. It is important to realise that technological advances inevitably come with benefits and risks. The international community has not yet developed effective regulatory instruments that may help to maximise benefits and minimise risks. As choices have to be made on the design and implementation of technological advances, these will need an assessment in terms of their contribution or damage to the protection of human dignity and security. Given the uncertainty of outcomes of the choices humans make, it is crucial to permanently and publicly discuss what motives guided decision-makers and whether choices can be accounted for as contributory to global respect of the right to health.

Questions for Discussion

- Discuss the advantages versus the disadvantages of an advanced digital database with all the patient personal data in your psychiatric institution.
- Discuss the terms of reference for the human rights assessment committee in your hospital.

References

Beck, U. (1992). *Risk society: Towards a new modernity*. Sage.

Nouri, A., & Chyba, C. F. (2008). Biotechnology and biosecurity. In N. Bostrom & M. M. Cirkovic (Eds.), *Global catastrophic risks* (pp. 450–480). Oxford University Press.

Winner, L. (1993). Citizen virtues in a technological order. In E. R. Winkler & J. R. Coombs (Eds.), *Applied ethics* (pp. 46–68). Basil Blackwell.

For Further Reading

Bostrom, N., & Cirkovic, M. M. (Eds.). (2008). *Global catastrophic risks*. Oxford University Press.

Brynjolfsson, E., & McAfee, A. (2015). *The second machine age*. Norton & Company.

Sterelny, K. (2012). *The evolved apprentice*. The MIT Press.

CHAPTER 13

Planning for the Future

Cees J. Hamelink, Dirk R. Essink and Marlies J. Visser

Introduction

Many of the moral choices that we have to make are made in uncertainty. However, we do not like uncertainty. A whole cottage industry of forecasters, sooth-sayers and prophets has emerged to offer us some certainty. The human obsession with certainty and completeness clashes with the difficult of planning for the future under conditions of uncertainty and ignorance. In this concluding chapter we want to discuss scenario planning as a possible way of dealing with and planning for the future. The scenario approach is inspired by a conversation in *Through the Looking Glass* where Alice says "I can't remember things before they happen", and the White Queen comments that "It's a poor sort of memory that only works backwards" (Lewis Carroll, 1865, p. 254). The White Queen can "remember the future" so that when the future happens she is not overwhelmed by surprise.

In the context of this book, anticipating planning for the future is critical as the authors aspire to an ongoing transformation to "a social and international order in which the rights and freedoms set forth in this Declaration can be fully realized" (Article 28, UDHR).

Learning Objectives

After studying this chapter you will be able to:

- See the future as multiple futures
- Deal with choices about the future as plausible stories about probable futures
- Apply the method of scenario development in concrete policy cases

The Future

Most of us are concerned about the future. We want to know what will happen next. We avidly read forecasts by experts on population explosions, climate change, imminent wars and economic crises. The future is important for us because, as Einstein once remarked,

DOI: 10.4324/9781003408765-17

"I intend to live in it!" The future is the only part of human life we can do something about. The past has gone and the present is as we speak already past. The future is the only dimension of human existence we can try to change. What most people find difficult about the future is the uncertainty it holds. In an increasingly complex world, we would prefer to have knowledge about what is in store for us, and we find it unsettling to admit that we are ignorant about the future. Therefore, we are inclined to make forecasts and to believe such forecasts, especially those that are produced by experts.

But can we actually forecast the future? Forecasting often departs from an inductivist base. It is guided by the assumption that one can make statements about the future on the basis of a limited number of past observations. Against inductivism, David Hume has proposed in his treatise on human nature (1739) that there is no logical argument for the conclusion that phenomena we have no knowledge about would resemble those we do know about. Inductivism has to assume an inherent continuity of the historical process. It forecasts the future with linear extrapolations based upon inductive reasoning. It needs to accept that history is a process of continuity and that there are unalterable laws of historical destiny. Such laws may be formulated by the physical sciences for the regularities in the physical environment, but there is no empirical indication that similar regularities are valid to the social environment.

Certainly, there are trends to be observed in human social history, but these are distinct from natural laws that determine the movement of a society and thus do not provide a valid prediction about society's future. Trends depend upon the specific configuration of historical conditions which themselves are not unequivocally determined. It is possible to establish correlations between trends and historical conditions, but these cannot in any way guarantee that a prediction based upon them is valid. Forecasts have a tendency to rely on expert opinions. However, this may be a risky business since predictions by experts are often wrong. Illustrative are the cases of Albert Einstein who was convinced (in 1932) that nuclear energy was impossible; of Thomas Alva Edison who claimed (in 1880) that the phonograph had no commercial value; of Lord Kelvin, the famous mathematician and president of the British Royal Society who announced (in 1878) that radio had absolutely no future or Paul Ehrlich's prediction of massive famines in the 1970s. One problem with experts is that they tend to be so confident about their opinions that they hardly listen to criticism and focus too much on one idea only. These are the experts that media love most:

> the sort who delivers quality sound bites and compelling stories. The sort who doesn't bother with complications, caveats, and uncertainties. The sort who has One Big idea. Yes, the sort of expert typically found in the media is most likely to be wrong.
>
> *(Garner, 2011, p. 27)*

In a rapidly changing world with uncertain futures, we need a vision of what the future might entail and what this means for human rights. What method could we use to base decisions upon (in politics, in business or in the military) that takes the future into account? One possibility is to write stories about plausible, possible futures. For decision-making in conditions of uncertainty, the scenario approach is a more useful tool than forecasting. The initiators of the scenario approach to the future were

Hermann Kahn and Gaston Berger. In the 1950s, Kahn developed stories for the US military about what would happen in case of a nuclear war between the US and the USSR. He called the "what-if" stories scenarios (Kahn, 1984). Gaston Berger, in Paris, created "La Prospective", a centre for future studies, and he designed normative scenarios for public policy. In his thinking, the future had to be invented as something new and unpredictable. The development of future scenario building really began in the 1960s and came into full swing in the 1970s when the emergence of the Organisation of the Petroleum Exporting Countries (OPEC) cartel and the environmentalism movement made future thinking particularly important for energy companies such as Shell.

Complex Adaptive Systems, Participation and Transition Management

Currently, visioning and scenario writing have gained prominence to address persistent problems within our complex adaptive systems. In particular, as the problems we face are often deeply entrenched in the system – often as negative side effects of positive elements in the systems – the logic of the past (forecasting) may not be useful to address problems of today. For example, within the energy system, carbon dioxide emission is a negative side effect of the great success of the fossil fuel-based energy system. And the lack of preventative services and preventative behaviour is likely a side effect of the successful cure-based health care system. Problem-solving in such a system is notoriously difficult and unpredictable, as i) these systems are path-dependent, implying that actors behave based on the rules and patterns laid out within the system, thereby reproducing the same problems within systems; ii) within change processes actors generally have different perceptions of the nature of the problem and they may critically differ regarding which facts, knowledge and values are deemed relevant when addressing problems within such systems; iii) external influences that affect the problem are hard to foresee (Loorbach, 2007).

These features make it hard to determine a course of action in change processes for reforming our systems to be more human rights based, as these processes are non-linear and their outcomes are highly unpredictable. Addressing these challenges often requires a systemic approach that considers the dynamics of the entire system. Therefore, simple trouble shooting and fixing problems in the present will not suffice. For a more profound systemic solution, we argue that a course of action should be based on back-casting[1] actions from a future vision, in other words, the narration of "scenarios".

Scenarios provide a structured way to explore different possible futures. Developing scenarios supports organisations and individuals to explore different potential outcomes, foresee risks and prepare for a range of possibilities, opportunities and threats. This enables decision-making and allows for a more robust strategy that can adapt to various future conditions. Within system innovation literature and transition management, scenario-writing is increasingly used to guide system change (Broerse & Grin, 2017). It is important to develop scenarios in participation with a range of actors who represent experts from different disciplines and societal sectors. It is critical to also include actors who are able to think beyond the current realities and practices. An example of this is the "transition arena", a conceptual space or platform where various stakeholders from academia, governments, business, civil society organisation and community members come together to engage in dialogue, collaboration and the co-creation of visions and strategies for guiding a societal transition (Notermans et al., 2022).

Scenarios are composed of plausible future states, based on different socio-technical trends or drivers, taking into account uncertainties related to behaviour of actors in the system. These socio-technical trends or drivers can, for example, relate to climate change, political changes (e.g., antidemocratic movements), conflict and/or AI. Scenarios are used to determine actions in the present to avoid worst-case scenarios and promote best-case scenarios.

The Method

Step 1: setting the scene. As a first step, participants in a scenario exercise will take stock of the work done in their field. They will discuss strengths versus weaknesses in past and current work and identify essential opportunities versus possible threats. Participants will also brainstorm about a timeline for the scenarios and identify trends/drivers and major uncertainties. Following this they will discuss and try to find a consensus about the key (political, economic, socio-cultural) variables for their scenarios. They decide on their preferred method of work; smaller groups; size; division of labour. Each working group (if it is decided to work in small teams) explores what empirical data need to be collected for their scenario(s) and how they will go about collecting those data.

Step 2: scenario development. As a second step, participants will actually build scenarios; design formats for presentation and present scenarios for public debate. A critical component of future scenarios is "backwards" planning. This means planning from the scenarios backwards to where we are today in order to explore what actions will have to be taken to avoid worst-case scenarios and what actions will have to be taken to achieve desirable future outcomes. Writing scenarios involves selecting key variables that are essential for future developments. These variables can be political, social, economic or cultural. This method enables the creation of structured and insightful scenarios that can aid in strategic planning and decision-making. A simple method for the writing of scenarios is the following:

- Selection of key variables: start with a thorough discussion and analysis to identify two key variables (these could be political, social, economic or cultural) that seem essential in future developments.
- Defining the horizontal and vertical axis: define each axis with two opposite realities of the selected variable articulated on each side of the axis (see Figure 13.1) – such as more political space for civil engagement versus less political space for civil engagement. Once these are set, four stories about possible futures emerge.
- Creating scenarios: the combination of these trends results in four quadrants, each representing a different story about possible futures. In each quadrant of the matrix the question is: what is the probable story if this combination of dimensions occurs?
- Identifying preferred futures: on the basis of the stories resulting from these questions, preferred versus undesirable futures can be identified. Preferred future scenarios describe desirable future outcomes. For these scenarios, the leading question is: if things went well, being optimistic but realistic, what would we see as desirable outcomes? It is important in this scenario to make underlying values and norms explicit and argue their relevance.

- Identifying undesirable futures: these are described as early warning scenarios and intended to assist in contingency planning. What plans must be prepared in case undesirable – even unlikely – outcomes are projected? For early warning scenarios, the leading question is: if things went wrong, what developments and outcomes would we worry about? It is important in these scenarios that the negative developments and outcomes are coherently argued.

A critical component of future scenarios is "backwards" planning. This means planning from the outcomes of the scenarios backwards to where we are today in order to explore what actions will have to be taken to avoid worst-case stories and what actions will have to be taken to achieve desirable future outcomes.

As an example, the future of human rights-based institutions for health care can be used. Selecting two important variables gives rise to four plausible scenarios (see Figure 13.1). For this example, we select the SDH as a variable in policy-making and put on the horizontal axis the two dimensions: low priority (i.e. SDH are not considered essential in health care policy) versus high priority (i.e. SDH are considered a priority in health care policy-making). On the vertical axis we may put the advancement of medical technology. The two dimensions are slow growth versus exponential growth.

It is of crucial importance to decide which variables to use for the two axes. This is the basis of the scenario exercise and you need all the creativity that participants can bring to the discussion to work this out. The task is to finish with a limited set of scenarios (usually four) that may contain guidance for future decision-making.

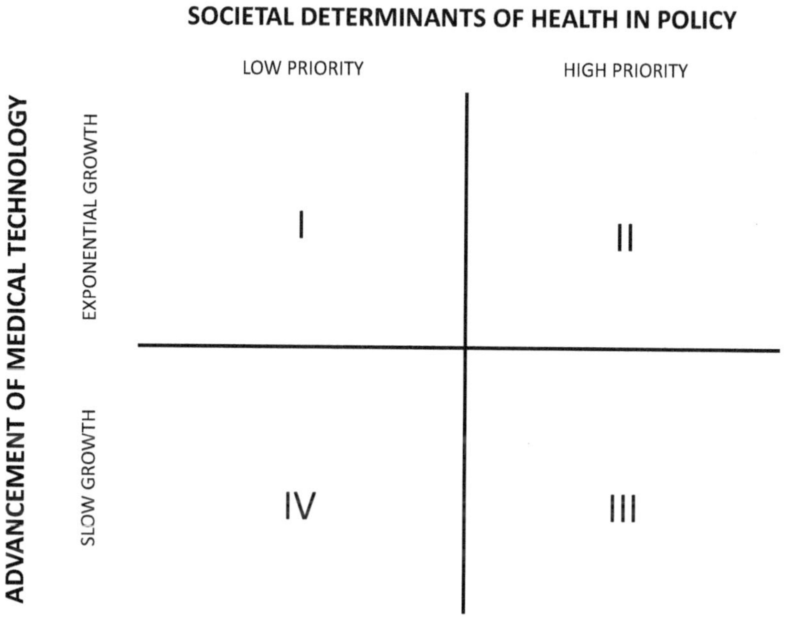

Figure 13.1 Societal Determinants of Health in Policy vs Advancement of Medical Technology

Writing the Scenarios

The literature on scenario building suggests incorporating elements of both desirable and undesirable futures within the different scenarios. There are four useful criteria that can help to write the scenarios:

1. Plausibility: the scenarios must be plausible; this means that they must fall within the limits of what might conceivably happen.
2. Consistency: the scenarios must be internally consistent. Inconsistent story lines erode the plausibility of the scenarios.
3. Relevance: the scenarios must be relevant to the focal issue defined at the beginning.
4. Challenge: the scenarios should contribute to new thinking about possible futures.

The scenarios have to be elaborated using descriptive titles, telling plausible and challenging stories, avoiding probabilities and using visual materials whenever possible to illustrate the stories in creative ways.

For a successful scenario exercise, it is important that participants take present situations and probable trends into account but liberate their minds from the temptation of forecasting. Participants should also realise that at its core the scenario approach is about "telling stories" to each other in an open and trusted environment and not about advancing parochial agendas. Scenario development is a creative and liberating exercise: it is fun but "serious fun" as it creates consciousness about emerging developments but also makes participants the co-authors of these developments. The best number of participants is 20–25, representing a broad variety of interests and professional backgrounds. Ideally, small teams of four or five participants work on the design, development and presentation of one scenario.

Implementing Scenarios

Scenarios can be used as a tool to create a framework for a shared vision of the future, to promote discussion and build consensus. Scenarios create awareness of thinking in uncertainties, and they widen horizons to reflect on how to deal with alternative plausible futures. The scenario exercise helps people start "seeing with new eyes" (Marcel Proust) and develop common ground for strategic conversations. Such conversations within organisations address the question of what strategic options can be seen in the different scenarios. These strategic conversations (fuelled by the scenarios) could become the daily conversations among members of an organisation with as basic requisites a common language, shared assumptions and values and the willingness to engage in dialogue.

Concluding Remarks

An effective and robust promotion and protection of human rights requires future planning. A host of demographic, institutional, political, economic and technological developments will affect the practice of health care. There will be both threats to fundamental rights and freedoms and chances for their realisation. We cannot forecast the future, but we can prepare for it through creating plausible stories about possible futures. As the White Queen tells us, "we can remember the future".

Questions for Discussion

- Select crucial variables pertinent to the future development of institutional health care. For example, variables relevant to future sexual and reproductive health care, care for children or disabled persons, elderly care or mental health care. Build four scenarios for decision-making and test them against human rights standards.
- Select crucial variables pertinent to realising Article 28 of the UDHR and build four scenarios for decision-making: "everyone is entitled to a social and international order in which the rights and freedoms set forth in this Declaration can be fully realised".

Note

1 Back-casting starts with a vision of a desired future state. Plan your actions from a desired vision. On the contrary, forecasting is basing decisions on current trends from historical data and building statistical models to design scenarios. Generally, forecasting is more relevant when the problems are less complex, interventions require systemic features similar to existing ones and outcomes can be more easily predicted. Back-casting is more useful when there is higher level of uncertainty. In practice, hybrid forms can be applied which involve back-casting from a desired future vision, taking into account current trends and insights.

References

Broerse, J., & Grin, J. (Eds.). (2017). *Toward sustainable transitions in healthcare systems.* Routledge.

Garner, D. (2011). *Future babble.* Penguin.

Kahn, H. (1984). *Thinking about the unthinkable in the 1980s.* Simon & Schuster.

Loorbach, D. (2007). *Transition management: New mode of governance for sustainable development.* International Books.

Notermans, I., von Wirth, T., & Loorbach, D. (2022). *An experiential guide for transition Arenas.* DRIFT, Erasmus University.

For Further Reading

Chermack, T. J. (2011). *Scenario planning in organizations.* Berrett-Koehler Publishers.

de Ruyter, P. (2016). *Scenario based strategy: Navigating the future.* Routledge.

Godet, M. (2006). *Creating futures: Scenario's planning as a strategic planning tool.* Economica.

Kahane, A. (2004). *Solving tough problems: An open way of talking, listening and creating new realities.* Berrett-Koehler Publishers.

Ringland, G. (1998). *Scenario planning: Managing for the future.* John Wiley & Sons.

Schwartz, P. (1991). *The art of the long view: Planning for the future in an uncertain world.* John Wiley & Sons.

van der Heijden, K. (1996). *Scenarios: The art of strategic conversation.* John Wiley & Sons.

Epilogue

We produced this book as a work in progress, fuelled by our ongoing interactions with students. The encounter of global health issues with the human rights framework is a story to be continued. We do indeed intend to do just that by listening to readers and especially to students who may want to include other topics, other dimensions and other approaches.

We will be happy to exchange thoughts with all those who want to contribute to an understanding of how we can enrich – worldwide – current and future practices and policies for healing and caring with the normative standards of international human rights.

Human rights are lived and can tell inspirational stories through which people can become agents of their own destinies. They are roadmaps towards just and equitable futures and also analytical tools to understand the root causes of injustice and inequity. The international human rights framework proposes a compassionate world inspired by dignity, freedom, equality and security. This is an imagination of a future world and a challenge to create human rights-based societies.

It is our conviction that meeting this challenge is a major step towards securing the human right to health for all people.

Index

AAAQ yardstick 1, 48, 89
access to technologies 204
Adami, R. 88
ADHD 124
Adhikari, S. 40
Afolab, A.B. 126
African Charter on Human and People's
    Rights 11, 92, 111
aging 149
Aikin, L.R. 156
Allan, D. 71
Alma Ata 46, 53
American Convention of Human Rights 11
American Declaration of Independence 9, 10
American Psychiatric Association 127
Americans with Disabilities Act 111
Amnesty International 7, 16, 47
Annan K. 9, 47
Apel, K.O. 73
Aristotle 71, 95
artificial intelligence 206
ASEAN Enabling Masterplan 111
autonomous patent 52, 53
Aziz Said, A. 23

back-casting 215
backwards planning 212
Baehr, P. 13
Barrett, D. 53
Beal, F. 99
Beck, U. 50, 203
Beijing Platform for Action 90

Bentham, J. 69
Berger, G. 211
bounded rationality 66, 186
Bradley, H. 50, 51
Brazilian Inclusion Law 111
Broerse, J. 211
Buber, M. 77

Carroll, L. 209
Castillo-Martell, H. 130
catastrophic health expenditure 36
CEDAW 15, 89
child soldier 140
Chios refugee camp 145
Christian theology 10
Chyba, C.F. 205
climate change 163
Collins, P.H. 99
colonialism 28, 161
colonial medicine 28
communication 77
community 76
complex adaptive systems 186, 211
Confucian culture 10
consequentialist method 70
Convention on the Rights of Persons with
    Disabilities 91, 110, 124, 130, 132, 157
Convention on the Rights of the Child 15, 90,
    135, 139, 140
Cook, R.J. 98
Coombs, J.R. 72
cosmovision 169

COVID-19 and Human Rights 187
Crenshaw, K. 99
cultural perceptions of aging 150
cultural perceptions of dying 156
cultural perceptions of mental
    health 125
culture 168
Current Challenges in Global Health 39
Cusack, S. 98
Cutipé-Cardenas, Y. 130

de Beauvoir, S. 81, 95
Déclaration des droits de l'homme et du
    citoyen 9, 10
Declaration of Independence 75
Declaration on the Rights of Mentally
    Retarded Persons 111
Declaration on the Use of Scientific and
    Technological Progress 202
Decolonising Global Health 40
deontology 67
derogations 183
Dewey, J. 137
diagnostics 126
dignity 8, 12, 13, 48, 50, 129, 155
disability 109
Disability Discrimination Act 111
disability-poverty cycle 116
discursive approach 73, 138
DSM-5 126
duration 21
Duska, R. 74
Dworkin, R. 20
Dyk, G.A. van 126

ECHR 7, 11, 52
ECOSOC 15
enforcement 14, 139
epistemic justice 40
equality 34, 47, 77
equity 33, 96, 183
ethical deep dialogue 78
ethics 66, 195
EU Charter of Fundamental Rights 91
eugenics 114
European Accessibility Act 111
European colonisation 161
European Court of Human Rights 139
Euthanasia 144
extractivism 163

food security 35, 177
forced treatment 124
Fraser, N. 137
Freire, P. 50
Fricker, M. 42
Fromm, E. 128
Fung, H.H. 151

Gandhi, M. 10
Garcia-Saya, D. 17
gender 94, 191
gender bias 96
gender stereotyping 98
Ghai, Y. 19
Gharner, D. 210
Gigerenzer, G. 75
Global Health 27, 31
Global Health Inequities 36
globalisation 19
Global North 40
Global South 40
Gostin, L.O. 44
Gouge, O.de 10
Greenhalgh, T. 194
Greenwood, A. 29
Grin, J. 211
Guthold, R. 136

Habermas, J. 73
Hague Convention 152
Haidt, J. 73
harmful effects 202
Harvard School of Public Health 47
health 30
Heise, L. 94
hermeneutical injustice 42
History of Global Health 28
Horton, R. 194
human choice 203
human mind 128
Human Rights Assessment 204
Human Rights Commission 14, 54, 139
Human Rights Council 56, 123
Human Rights Education 55, 56
Human Rights Ethics 65
Human Rights Watch 7, 47

ICCPR 11, 14, 15, 89, 152
ICPD 85
ICSER 11, 16, 46, 110, 152, 180
IMF 16
impairment 109
imperialism 28
Indigenous knowledge 28, 169
Indigenous populations 28, 161, 170
Individuals with Disabilities Education
    Act 111
inequality 49
informed consent 205
institutional choices 79
Inter-American Commission on Human
    Rights 164, 167
Inter-American Human Rights
    Court 131
International Classification of Functioning,
    Disability and Health (ICF) 114

International Federation of Human
    Rights 7
international health 29
International Health Regulations 31, 180
intersectionality 32, 99, 114
intuitionism 73
Islamic Declaration of Human Rights 11
Islamic theology 10
Istanbul Convention 91

Jongman, J. J. 13
Joy, A.O. 126
justice 34
justiciability 21
justification 7, 75

Kahn, H. 211
Kant, I. 8
Kanter, A.S. 157
Keizer, B. 153
Koplan, J. 32
Kumar, R. 41
Küme Mogen (balance in health) 171

League of Nations 9, 135
liberty 48, 77
Limitations and Derogations 183
Lipman. M. 137
Locke, J. 8, 9
Loorbach, D. 211
Lorde, A. 99

MacIntyre, A. 71
Magna Carta 9
Mann, J. 47
the Maputo Protocol 92
Masquelier, B. 136
maternal mortality 93
medical genetics 205
medical model of disability 112
mental health 123
Millennium Development Goals 54, 55
Mill, J.S. 69
moral choice 65, 209
morality 66
moral obligation 9, 67

Naidu, T. 42
An Na'im, A. 19
Nefale, M. 126
normalcy 109
Notermans, I. 211
Nouri, A. 205

Ogé V. 10
OPEC 211
Os, J. van 127
Othering 81

Paine, T. 10
palliative sedation 154
pandemics 184
Partsch, K.J. 14
Perin, J. 136
Perrucci, R. 51
planetary health 31, 177
planning 209
Plato 136
power 50
proportionality 21
PTSD 144
public health 29
Public Health Emergency of International
    Concern (PHEIC) 179
public sphere 138

Qu'ran 19

Rahman, M. 132
Rawls, J. 138
reason 75
reproductive health and rights 85
right to health 30, 45, 47, 88, 135, 141, 149,
    179, 201
Rivera-Holguin, M. 130
Roosevelt, F.D. 12

Said, E. 81
Santa Barbara Massacre 131
scenario approach 210
Schmidt, A.P. 13
security 48, 77
Sedgwick, H. 70, 73, 75
sense-making 76
Sepur Zarco Case 131
sexual and reproductive health and rights 85
Shari'a 19
Siracusa Principles 184
social conditionalities 48
social determinants of health 30
social intuition model 73
social model of disability 112
social rights 117
societal barriers to human rights for disabled
    people 117
Sommer, C. 74
Sommer, F. 74
Sousa, R. de 80
state obligation 16
state sovereignty 7
subsidiarity 21
Sustainable Development Goals (SDGs)
    35, 91

technology 201
Teheran Conference on Human Rights 201
testimonial injustice 42

third generation 13
Thys, W. 76
Tibbits, F. 57
Tobin, J. 52, 53
Toyama, M. 130
transition management 211
tropical medicine 32

UDHR 7, 9, 11, 20, 23, 46, 57, 65, 75, 88,
    110, 136, 141, 151, 201, 209, 215
UN Charter 9, 11, 29
UN Commission on the Status of Women 88
UN Decade of Healthy Aging 150
UN Declaration on the Rights of Indigenous
    Peoples 166
UNESCO 10
UNFPA 47
UNICEF 140
Universal Declaration of Human
    Responsibilities 25, 57
Universal Health Coverage 31, 35, 53
UN Security Council 17

UN Special Rapporteurs 47, 54, 56, 123
UN World Conference on Human Rights 15,
    22, 139
urbanisation 49
utilitarian method 69

vaccine inequality 192
Velazquez, T. 130
Vienna Declaration and Platform for Action
    22, 90
virtue-based method of ethics 71

white supremacy 161
WHO 29, 45, 53, 123, 136, 150, 180
Winkler, E.R. 72
Winner, L. 204
World Assembly on Aging 151
World Inequality Report 51
World Report on Aging and Health 158
Wysing, E. 5

Zidar, A. 183